ETHICS
IN REHABILITATION

A Clinical Perspective

ETHICS
IN REHABILITATION

A Clinical Perspective

Barbara L. Kornblau, JD, OT/L, FAOTA, DAAPM, ABDA, CDSM, CCM
Shirley P. Starling, JD, MHS

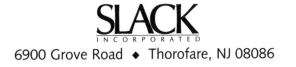
SLACK
INCORPORATED
6900 Grove Road ◆ Thorofare, NJ 08086

Publisher: John H. Bond
Editorial Director: Amy E. Drummond
Associate Editor: Jennifer L. Stewart

The work SLACK Incorporated publishes is peer reviewed. Prior to publication, recognized leaders in the field, educators, and clinicians provide important feedback on the concepts and content that we publish. We welcome feedback on this work.

Kornblau, Barbara.
    Ethics in rehabilitation: a clinical perspective / Barbara Kornblau, Shirley Starling.
        p. cm.
    Includes bibliographical references and index.
    ISBN 1-55642-353-5 (alk. paper).
    1. Medical rehabilitation--Moral and ethical aspects. 2. Rehabilitation--Law and legislation--United States.

RM930 .K67 1999
174'.2--dc21

99-053933

Printed in the United States of America.
Published by: SLACK Incorporated
                 6900 Grove Road
                 Thorofare, NJ 08086-9447 USA
                 Telephone: 856-848-1000
                 Fax: 856-853-5991
                 www.slackinc.com

Contact SLACK Incorporated for more information about other books in this field or about the availability of our books from distributors outside the United States.

Last digit is print number: 10 9 8 7 6 5 4 3 2 1

DEDICATION

This book is dedicated to the loving memory of Austin Neal Wyrick,
an ethical man in word and deed.

CONTENTS

Section I. Approaches to Ethical Dilemmas

Section II. Ethical Dilemmas: Practical Applications

Section III. Ethical Dilemma Worksheets

Section IV. Appendices

ACKNOWLEDGMENTS

This book celebrates a collaboration of two occupational therapist-attorneys and hopefully answers the question, "What does law have to do with occupational therapy?" once and for all.

Over the years, we have found ethical dilemmas in our own clinical practices, as well as those of coworkers, students, and faculty colleagues. Barbara receives many letters, e-mails, and telephone calls from therapists facing ethical dilemmas. All of these occupational therapy colleagues have contributed to the making of this book in one way or another, and we thank them.

We also thank our colleagues on the occupational therapy faculty at Nova Southeastern University for their encouragement and assistance while we wrote this book. We especially thank Dr. Reba Anderson for her motivation and inspiration; Dr. Lori Andersen for her invaluable assistance in reading drafts along the way, making invaluable, pain-free suggestions, and coming up with the acronym "CELIBATE"; and Dr. Rosalie Miller for answering questions on becoming a book author.

We are grateful to the present and former occupational therapy doctoral students at Nova Southeastern University—among them Robinette J. Strutton-Amaker, Major, US Army, Dr.OT, MHE, OTR/L; Wendy Kaplan, BS, OTR; and Elyse Lipschultz, MS, OTR/L—for their contribution of ethical dilemmas, and to our masters level students who shared ethical dilemmas with us and helped us field test and refine our methodology.

We thank Marcia Colmar, MA, OTR/L for graciously sharing her knowledge of Medicare regulations and for her assistance in gathering other Medicare sources of information from the Internet, and E.J. Brown, Editor, *Advance for Occupational Practitioners*, for participating in numerous discussions regarding ethical issues and the current state of practice.

Barbara thanks her mentors, in particular Dr. Judith Leavitt, for teaching her to consider the significance of the historical perspective in health care and who, together with Linda Anderson, MS, OTR, FAOTA, Melanie Ellexson, MBA, OTR, FAOTA, Cynthia Epstein, MA, OTR, FAOTA, Jean Kiernat, MS, OTR, FAOTA, Joane Wyrick, MS, OTR, FAOTA, and countless others, helped her develop as an ethical practitioner and encouraged her to pursue her dreams.

Barbara also thanks her husband, Larry Sherry, who has attended more occupational therapy conferences than have most practicing occupational therapists, and her six children, Allan, Paula, Mindy, Logan, Stephanie, and Vito, for their contributions.

We are indebted to all the people at SLACK Incorporated for their patience and support, and without whom this book would not have been possible.

Above all, we thank the students over the years who have taught us about ethical dilemmas in their lives, as well as all the anonymous people who have written and called with ethical dilemmas.

About the Authors

Barbara L. Kornblau, JD, OT/L, FAOTA, DAAPM, ABDA, CDSM, CCM, is a professor of occupational therapy and public health at Nova Southeastern University, North Miami Beach, FL. In her private practice, she provides consulting services to business and industry, attorneys, and others. A practicing attorney, she specializes in disability discrimination and related issues. A graduate of the University of Wisconsin-Madison and the University of Miami School of Law, she has published numerous journal articles, book chapters, and other works on the Americans With Disabilities Act, medical-legal issues, ethics, consultation, and work rehabilitation.

Shirley P. Starling, JD, MHS, is an attorney in private practice in Fort Lauderdale, FL. Ms. Starling received her Bachelor of Science and Master of Health Science degrees in occupational therapy at the University of Florida, and her Juris Doctorate degree at Nova Southeastern University. She has 25 years of experience as an occupational therapist in mental health and served on the faculty of the undergraduate program at Florida International University and the graduate program at Nova Southeastern University. She has provided professional and community educational programs on both occupational therapy and legal issues.

INTRODUCTION

The concept for this book developed as the authors found themselves fielding, with increasing frequency, questions from students and practicing clinicians about ethical and related legal dilemmas in clinical rehabilitation practice. The changing trends in health care seemed to provide additional challenges to practitioners and, thus, this book was born.

The authors present rehabilitation practitioners with practical information about ethics from a clinical perspective. The book is organized to give rehabilitation professionals the knowledge and tools they need to solve the ethical dilemmas that challenge them today and an opportunity to apply the information they acquire. Following an introduction to ethical theories and ethical principles, the first section furnishes readers with a brief overview of legal principles that may impact on ethical decision-making, then examines the relationship between ethical and legal principles that clinicians may encounter in everyday practice. In Section I, the authors also present a system that rehabilitation practitioners may use to analyze and solve ethical dilemmas.

Section II provides readers with an opportunity to apply what they have learned to 115 sample ethical dilemmas extracted from actual practice experiences. The ethical dilemmas cover a wide variety of practice-related topics that each apply to several professions within the rehabilitation arena.

In Section III, readers will find an extensive appendix with samples codes of ethics, sample laws and regulations, as well as an extensive list of internet resources. Readers can use these resources to assist them in examining and solving the ethical dilemmas. The internet resources include links to websites where readers may find full-text versions of their own state licensure laws and related laws as well as regulations that may impact ethical practice.

Our purpose is to offer readers a practical approach to ethics within a clinical context to allow practitioners to raise questions, attempt to answer them, and promote and improve ethical practice in rehabilitation.

Approaches to Ethical Dilemmas

1

Introduction

When we began practicing occupational therapy in the 1970s, we treated patients until "they were better"; in other words, until the rehabilitation team—consisting of occupational, physical, and speech therapy; social work; and nursing (with a little input from the patient's physician)—"felt" the patients no longer needed our intervention. Without pressure to discharge patients, therapy practitioners treated patients until the patients no longer needed us or their insurance ran out, which often gave patients and therapists several months of intensive inpatient treatment together. Patients simply received more time in therapy to reach the highest level of ability possible before discharge.

At the same time, the reverse proved true to some extent. In some cases, patients with poor prognoses received treatment with minimal apparent benefit. Insurance paid for the services and the "treaters" could meet the bottom line "to help people and make money"—the two being not mutually exclusive and easily accomplishable together as one goal.

Together with our colleagues, we looked at "ethics" as a theoretical concept studied in school that experienced minimal application in clinical, educational, or fieldwork practice. Boy, have things changed!

Over the last several years, we saw an increase in overutilization of services in rehabilitation and a stern response by payers to limit reimbursement. We saw patients discharged from inpatient settings often before they were ready to face the demands outside the hospital. Fraudulent billing practices lurked in the shadows along with treatment by unqualified personnel, documentation irregularities, and the pressure of other questionable practices.

WHY STUDY ETHICS?

"My belief is that no human being or society composed of human beings ever did or ever will come to much unless their conduct was governed and guided by the love of some ethical ideal."
Thomas H. Huxley, quoted in Seldes, 1972

"Why study ethics?" some clinicians, educators, administrators, supervisors, and students have asked. They may add: "If I go to work every day, do my job, and mind my own business, I don't need to worry about ethics." Or: "I've been a practicing therapy professional for 20 years. Why do I need to worry about ethics now?"

Ethics Defined

The American Heritage Dictionary defines an *ethic* as "A principle of right or good conduct or a body of such principles" and *ethics* as "The study of the general nature of morals and of specific moral choices." Some consider ethics the study of right and just behavior and choices. In our personal lives, we face moral problems to which we must respond by making specific moral choices. The specific moral choice one makes will undoubtedly vary from person to person based on a number of factors, ranging from religious and cultural influences to one's individual value system.

Foundation of Ethics and Ethical Conflict

Whereas one's study of ethics may begin here with these pages, shaping of ethics, values, and morals begins in childhood as our morals, values, and religious beliefs form a foundation for us. During our maturation process, we pick and choose the morals, values, and beliefs we wish to incorporate into our own belief system from those taught to us. We have an opportunity to make choices as to how we wish others to perceive us. We can also choose those values that form a basis for the reputation we desire as we develop as individuals. What do we want others to think of our reputations and ourselves? Certainly, our choices affect our relationships with others as we develop.

Children learn early in life where they fit in relation to a pecking order of authorities. Various contributions from these authorities contribute to their ethics and morals. Some children are tempted to let these "authorities" make their decisions rather than think for themselves. Who are these authorities?

1. **Social norms**. The first type of authority is the dictates of social norms. Children learn to respect the authority of social norms, traditions, cultures, and customs. As they develop, children and adolescents learn what is expected of them and what is proper. In response to "Why can't I do that?" the child may hear "That's just not done," "This is how we do it," or "We've always done it this way."

2. **Authority figures**. The second type of authority includes teachers, bosses, leaders, and other authority figures who possess power over children and adolescents and, in the process, command respect. As children and adolescents face more and more "have-to's" in their lives, they learn to respect those who give them orders.

3. **Religious orientation**. The third authority, stemming from one's religious orientation, is a higher power. Most children learn to respect a higher power and the teachings of a particular religious orientation to which they may look for definitive moral rules. Religious doctrines provide some commonly known lessons, which for some provide the basis for their morals and ethics. The golden rule, "Do unto others as you would have them do unto you," finds roots in both the Old Testament and the New Testament of the Bible as well as other holy books and writings from other religions. All religions have their own similar standard (Table 1-1). Franklin D. Roosevelt told his own version of the golden rule: "If you treat people right they will treat you right—90% of the time" (quoted in Baker, 1992).

4. **Traditional popular culture**. Many of us grew up with expressions and phrases parents or other adults quoted to us at times they felt we needed to learn a lesson about life. These expressions add to the ethical foundation of the individual. Phrases such as "Honesty is the best policy," "Two wrongs don't make a right," "Never put off until tomorrow what you can do today," "If you can't say something good about a person, don't say anything at all," and "It's not whether you win or lose, but how you play the game" become part of our belief system.

5. **Contemporary popular culture**. Popular culture gives us "buzzword ethics." Buzzword ethics—usually hollow words popularized by an advertisement or song—attract many. Phrases can be entwined so tightly into popular culture that they often play a significant role in the formation of one's ethical foundation. Individuals often look to these phrases when they seek choices and answers (Table 1-2).

Developing a sense of ethics requires that an individual pick and choose from the value lessons learned in life and develop independent thinking abilities.

Table 1-1

The Golden Rule in Major Religions

RELIGION	STATEMENT	SOURCE
Judaism	Thou shalt not avenge nor bear any grudge against the children of thy people, but thou shalt love thy neighbor as thyself: I am the Lord.	Leviticus 19:18
	What is hateful to you, do not do to your fellow men. That is the entire law; all the rest is commentary.	Talmud: Shabbat 31a
Islam	No one of you is a believer until he desires for his brother what which he desires for himself.	Sunnah
Christianity	All things, therefore, that you want men to do to you, you also must likewise do to them, for this is the law.	Matthew 7:12
Buddhism	Hurt not others in ways that you yourself would find hurtful.	Udana-Varga 5:18
Confucianism	Surely it is the maxim of loving-kindness: Do not unto others that you would not have them do unto you.	Analects 15, 23
Taoism	Regard your neighbor's gain as your own gain, and your neighbor's loss as your own loss.	T'ai Shang Kan Ying P'ien
Brahmanism	This is the sum of duty: Do naught unto others which would cause you pain if done to you.	Mahabharta 5, 1517

Table 1-2

Popular Culture's "Buzzword Ethics"

SLOGAN	SOURCE
"Just do it"	Nike
"I think I can ... I think I can"	The Little Engine that Could
"Have it your way"	Burger King
"Don't Worry-Be Happy"	Bobby McFerron
"Think Different"	Apple Computer
"I'll make him an offer he can't refuse"	Mario Puzo and Vito Corleone

ETHICAL CONFLICTS

When values conflict, or "shoulds," "coulds," and "should nots" stand in the way of acting, absent an internal struggle, individuals may face an ethical dilemma. For example, individuals may face a situation knowing they "could" choose a particular course of action but probably "should" chose a different one, and definitely "should not" choose a third option.

A dilemma is a choice between two equally compelling alternatives—a predicament for which one finds no singular or clear-cut satisfactory solution. An ethical dilemma requires a choice between equally compelling values. Health professionals face ethical dilemmas when in the course of competent practice they see severe harm at stake or benefits in jeopardy no matter what course of action they take (Erde, 1998). In other words, when a situation arises where one's response or actions can cause negative consequences or nullify the benefits of good consequences, one has an ethical dilemma.

Many factors influence how an individual both perceives and resolves an ethical dilemma. Personal life experience (or lack thereof), by the incorporation of social values, moral principles, religious training, and cultural factors, influences an individual's ethical values.

The nature of an ethical choice influences its resolution. One can view an ethical conflict from three perspectives: personal, organizational, or societal. These perspectives are not mutually exclusive. Any one ethical problem requires consideration of each perspective.

A personal dilemma involves concern for the

good of the individual. In health care, a personal dilemma may involve a choice between respecting a patient's right to privacy and the professional's need to know information in order to treat the patient appropriately.

An organizational dilemma involves issues affecting an institution such as a hospital, professional association, business, or family. Health care professionals often find themselves asked to act to benefit the organization (hospital) in a way that may compromise benefit to the individual (patient).

The third perspective—societal—places emphasis on the well-being of the community or society as a whole. The historical decision to isolate persons with Hanson's disease (leprosy) from the rest of the community exemplifies a resolution using this perspective.

A health professional faced with an ethical dilemma will quickly realize that the values in question go beyond professional values to include personal values. Individuals may find their personal values deeply ingrained and quickly asserted. One's personal values may result in emotional responses or failure to consider other perspectives, generate alternatives, or consider the needs or position of others involved in the situation. In the professional arena, one must acknowledge personal values and, once acknowledged, one must explore alternate values and issues.

For example, suppose one treats a patient who is near death and, in fact, is not expected to live for more than 2 weeks. The professional knows the patient possesses a living will, which states that if the patient is terminally ill with no possibility of recovery, the patient wants no active treatment of any kind except medication to relieve pain. As a resident in a skilled nursing facility, the patient must receive skilled care in order to remain in the facility. The patient who lives alone and has no family cannot safely return home due to the extent of illness. As the only professional on staff and the only person who can provide skilled care for the patient, what will the therapy professional do?

What types of choices will affect decision-making in this situation? Personal value choices? Professional value choices? How many perspectives are considered in reaching an initial conclusion about a course of action?

Boy, Have Things Changed!

Ethical dilemmas have always played a role in the professional lives of health professionals. In today's world, we continue to witness a surge of interest in ethics and ethical principles. Judging from the recently emerging concerns of health care professionals, the number, quality, and tenor of these ethical struggles have changed in recent years and, consequently, the quest for answers and solutions broadens.

Why have these ethical struggles reached such a crescendo? Many reasons exist for the change. One can point to many factors for the answer to this question, but managed care probably stands out as the most significant role in turning the tide for health professionals.

Managed Care

Managed care has forced drastic changes in the health care system, many of which force ethical questions to the surface. Managed care has engendered many changes for health care practitioners. For example, occupational and physical therapy personnel face the threat of drives to cross-train with a variety of other allied health professionals as a way of keeping costs down for hospitals. Therapy practitioners continue to see increasing caseloads in an effort to do more with less, creating circumstances that make them question their ability to provide adequate care. Many face the increasing utilization of aides or rehab techs, and the pressure to use these unlicensed professionals under questionable circumstances. Capitation in rehabilitation and long-term care—the payment of a lump sum to cover all rehabilitation services—causes conflicts among the providers of therapy services over the often paltry amount of money that does not even cover one service's charges. This competition for dollars enhances the pressure to provide therapy services in the cheapest way possible: using aides or rehabilitation technicians. Readers will find more in-depth information about ethics and managed care in Chapter 4.

Managed care's decreased reimbursement has led to other problems, which by themselves also raise ethical concerns. Corporate downsizing and corporate mergers, often directly attributable to pressures from managed care, force layoffs of experienced managers and shifting responsibilities. The shift to program management—forming treatment teams based on the program (e.g., pediatrics or neurology) as opposed to departmentalization (e.g., occupational therapy or speech language pathology)—shifts practitioners from one field to a position of supervision over practitioners in another field. Less experienced subordinate employees seeking mentors may find their needs unmet by supervisors from other professions. The resulting lack of mentorship opportunities within the individual's profession changes the way professionals develop, especially with entry-level and young therapists, and may eliminate some growth opportunities. Supervisors from different professions often lack knowledge of their subordinate employees' codes of ethics and standards of practice, ordering those employees to perform questionable professional actions.

Changing Regulations

"The trouble with our times is that the future is not what it used to be."
Paul Valery, quoted in Gardner & Reese, 1996

Rapid changes in regulations governing health care and the accompanying confusion also contribute to the rise in ethical dilemmas. Over time, as these changes occurred, referrals seemed driven by reimbursement as opposed to patient needs. The institution of salary equivalency rules in physical therapy and speech pathology caused a shift in long-term care referrals to occupational therapy, initially exempt from salary equivalency. Once the federal government announced its intention to include occupational therapy under the salary equivalency rules, panic set in. By the time therapy professionals figured out a response to the salary equivalency rule, the government passed new regulations making the prospective payment system the law and salary equivalency meaningless.

The prospective payment system in long-term care opened yet another door of concern. Some fear the pressure to cut therapy billings under the prospective pay system may lead clinicians down the path of ethical dilemmas. These systems, designed to decrease fraud and abuse, will undoubtedly lead some clever administrators to "find a way around them." These schemes may tempt some therapists.

Uncertainty about job security accompanied the introduction of the prospective payment system. For the first time, therapists found themselves facing layoffs and difficulties obtaining employment. This additional factor may influence the incidence of ethical dilemmas by increasing competition among professionals seeking to perform within the scope of other professionals' domains, as well as competition with lesser qualified personnel such as aides and techs.

Cultural Diversity

Another factor contributing to the increase in ethical dilemmas in practice is cultural diversity. In past eras, we lived and worked in communities with individuals whose backgrounds mirrored our own. Similar religious, ethnic, and socioeconomic backgrounds often produced similar values. In recent years, new waves of immigrants coming from many sources around the globe have stirred the melting pot and injected society with a new dose of cultural diversity. Therapy practitioners may no longer assume ease of communication with a patient when language or cultural differences exist. The influx of foreign-trained therapists and other health practitioners increases the cultural diversity of coworkers, as well as patients and family members.

Cultural diversity also includes students and therapy practitioners with disabilities. IDEA (Individuals with Disabilities Education Act, formerly referred to as Public Law 94-142) requires public schools to provide free and appropriate education to individuals with disabilities. Now the Americans with Disabilities Act (ADA) seeks to eliminate discrimination in the workplace as well as in places of public accommodation such as schools and hospitals. The ADA also gives qualified individuals with disabilities rights to reasonable accommodations in the workplace to enable them to work. The ADA provides the right of reasonable accommodation to enable individuals to complete higher education programs and participate in programs offered by places of public accommodation. Students and practitioners with disabilities find themselves working side by side with nondisabled practitioners. Therapy practitioners may face difficulties dealing not only with patients or coworkers from other cultures based on ethic differences but also with individuals with disabilities. Some therapy practitioners find it easier to relate to individuals with disabilities as patients rather than peers.

Changing Societal Values

The proliferation of ethical dilemmas also stems from changes in society's values as a whole. The junk bond scandal of the 1980s, the "me" generation, the inability to accept delayed gratification, the increase in incidents of cheating on college campuses, the break-up of the family, and the quest for material wealth all change the focus from people to possessions. As money becomes the ultimate value, the quest for more money justifies behavior previously thought to be unacceptable.

Changing Political Values

"Where there is a lack of morals in government, the morals of the whole people are poisoned."
Herbert Hoover, quoted in Baker, 1992

Ethical issues in politics capture popular conversation. Political scandals reaching from local politics all the way up to the presidency make people question their belief systems. In Miami, FL, dead people occupying cemetery plots located outside the city limits voted en masse by absentee ballot in the mayoral election. After serving time for a cocaine conviction, Marion Barry was re-elected mayor by the people of the District of Columbia. For many months, a glance at any newspaper headline gave details about President Clinton's extramarital affair. Many agree that something is wrong when leadership and morality do not go hand in hand.

Technological Advances

Technological advances contribute to ethical struggles. Scientific advances constantly create myriad opportunities for the use or misuse of concepts and technology. People now survive serious accidents and illnesses once thought hopeless and live longer because of advances in medical technology, but sometimes the ethics surrounding these advances are hazy. Once the subject of science fiction, cloning, frozen embryos, and genetic mapping have entered the mainstream, and they come with a potentially high ethical cost.

Limited Resources

Limited resources contribute to compromised ethics. Limited resources remind society that it has yet to answer the question: "Is health care a right or a privilege?" Although new discoveries in medicine continue to spew more technology and costly medications into the health care arena, who can afford them? Will insurance companies pay for first-rate care inventions? Who will fund their development?

The Information Age

Easy access to information threatens ethical standards. We live in an age where consumers can instantly access information on the Internet. Consumers also may educate themselves by reading or watching television. In this information age, as therapists and members of the health care community, we find ourselves before more educated consumers who demand more of us and seem constantly to seek more information. Information is disseminated quickly. Patients question everything. "Don't worry. Medicare will pay for it" no longer satisfies the educated, information-age consumer.

The information age has changed the way we conduct ourselves and has invaded our patients' privacy. Students can access term papers on the Web, allowing term paper scandals on college campuses. Health care providers have always questioned the sanctity of paper documentation, and now computers threaten confidentiality even more. Computers can access a plethora of information about one's past, possibly discovering secrets not intended for public consumption. Within a hospital exists the possibility of accessing personal data about a patient's life, and sometimes that information can accidentally escape our best efforts of confidentiality. The Clinton administration's suggestion of health care identification numbers set off a frenzy of complaints by citizens concerned about their privacy, causing the administration to pause and rethink its strategy.

SUMMARY

The proliferation of ethical dilemmas seems to have created a crisis in therapy. A sense of panic envelops some therapy practitioners who do not know where to turn. Still others do not recognize an ethical problem when it exists.

Practicing therapists facing unfamiliar territory look for answers. When faced with an ethical problem or dilemma arising in the practice of therapy, therapists must figure out what to do about the dilemma. They need to answer questions that arise during the course of trying to solve a dilemma.

Clinicians, educators, administrators, supervisors, and students must learn the realities of ethical practice. Although studying ethical theory gives one the basis from which to make a judgment about a particular "problem," it does not provide the basis upon which to formulate a solution. It may raise more questions and fail to answer those questions. Merely making a judgment about the ethical dilemma one faces fails as a response to the dilemma. Practicing clinicians, educators, administrators, supervisors, and students need tools to translate their judgments into specific action steps to solve ethical dilemmas.

The authors cannot articulate a specific test to teach readers to identify each and every time they face an ethical dilemma. This determination relies on one's own analysis of conflicts among one's own morals, values, and beliefs. The authors hope that as readers begin to feel comfortable analyzing some of the ethical dilemmas in this book, they will find it easier to identify additional ethical dilemmas as they occur.

REFERENCES

Baker, D. B. (1992). *Power quotes.* Detroit, MI: Visible Ink Press.

Erde, E. L. (1998). A method of ethical decision making. In J. F. Monagle & D. C. Thomasma. (Eds.). *Health care ethics.* Gaithersburg, MD: Aspen.

Gardner, J. W., & Reese, F. G. (1996). *Wit & wisdom.* WW Norton & Company.

Seldes, G. (1972). *The great quotations.* New York: Simon & Schuster.

2

Ethics: The Basics

"Always do right. This will gratify some people and astonish the rest."
Mark Twain, *quoted in Gardner & Reese,1996*

Very simply stated, ethics guide the determination of right and wrong in moral life. Health and rehabilitation professionals must come to terms with moral issues in their lives to make choices in situations that arise in practice. However, before one can delve into ethical issues, one must examine ethical theories, terminology, and concepts to develop an understanding upon which to base further analysis of specific situations one may encounter.

TYPES OF ETHICAL THEORY

Ethical theories or theories of moral obligations give us a justification for ethical decision making. Several broad theories are presented to give readers a look at formal methods of ethical decision making.

Consequentialism or Teleological Theory

Consequentialism, or teleological theory, focuses on consequences and outcomes of a deed or action in answering the question, "What should I do?" (Shannon, 1997). The individual judges the "goodness" or "badness" of his or her ultimate decision by responding to the question, "Which action will produce the best outcome?" Where no clear answer emerges, this theory tells us to choose the course of

action that brings the most good and the least harm (Graber, 1998). People who subscribe to this theory approve of paternalistic behavior as long as one ultimately benefits from the action and no one gets hurt (Gert, Culver, & Clouser, 1997).

Deontologism Theory

Deontologism theory focuses not on the consequences of an action but on the type of action, and whether the action follows moral rules and principles. Those who follow the deontologism theory focus on one's duty or obligations in order to determine an ethical course of action. This theory focuses on strictly following rules and principles of ethics, such as respect for autonomy, nonmaleficence, beneficence, justice, and other moral factors previously discussed. The Ten Commandments exemplify a deontologic approach to ethics (Shannon, 1997).

Rights-Based Ethics

Rights-based ethics look to a person's individual rights in making ethical choices for a course of action. These rights can include legal rights, ethical rights, and political rights (Beauchamp & Childress, 1994). To solve ethical dilemmas under this theory, one must determine what rights the individual possesses. For example, those on both sides of the abortion debate—right to choice versus right to life—promote their beliefs using a rights-based approach to ethics (Shannon, 1997).

Virtue or Character-Based Ethics

"Character is much easier kept than recovered."
Thomas Paine, quoted in Gardner & Reese, 1996

Virtue, or character-based, ethics concerns itself with the types of virtues, integrity, or character traits one should display. This theory examines the roles one plays and the behavioral expectations each role encourages or requires. The individual can choose a course of action based on his or her role and the expectations that conform with that role. When conflicts occur, one chooses the course of action that allows him or her to embody the most moral character traits (Sim, 1997). Will Rogers gave an example of virtue or character-based ethics when he said, "I'd rather be the man who bought the Brooklyn Bridge than the man who sold it" (Peter, 1977).

Intuitionism-Based Ethics

Those who follow intuitionism-based ethical theory solve ethical dilemmas by following their intuition to determine right action from wrong action. One's moral sense takes over and allows the person to justify his or her action because, "the fact that I know something is right justifies my doing it" (Shannon, 1997). Intuitionism allows us to follow our convictions but ignores the need to deal with the contradictory opinions of others or to win them over to our own side.

Casuistry or Case-Based Ethics

Casuistry or case-based reasoning looks to the facts of specific cases to find solutions for ethical dilemmas. The casuistry approach uses a practical, case-based approach to apply abstract principles such as moral duties to specific sets of facts or cases. This approach looks to other similar cases as precedents to determine which rules best apply and which interpretation of the rules best suits the specific facts of the case (Gert, Culver, & Clouser, 1997). Some

refer to this approach as "applied ethics" (Arras, 1998). Precedence plays an important role, as does reasoning from other similar situations (Beauchamp & Childress, 1994).

BASIC PRINCIPLES OF ETHICS

Many books on ethics focus heavily on formal principles of ethics and ethical theories as a springboard to making ethical choices and solving ethical dilemmas. Although the authors take a slightly different approach to ethical decision making, a review of basic ethics terminology will contribute to the reader's understanding and broaden the reader's perspective on ethical principles and thought.

Autonomy

Autonomy refers to one's moral right to make choices and decisions about one's own course of action, in other words, the right to self-determination (Monagle, 1998). American society promotes autonomy in social, legal, and ethical circles. In the Declaration of Independence, the founding fathers affirmed the individual's entitlement to autonomy in its declaration of "life, liberty, and the pursuit of happiness."

Respect for autonomy dictates that one refrain from interfering with the individual's own choices (Jonsen, Seigler, & Winslade, 1998). The principle of autonomy assumes one's ability to analyze alternatives, make a responsible choice, and carry out one's plans. For example, an individual who lives in a persistive vegetative state following an accident cannot analyze alternatives, make a choice, or carry out plans or actions. One may ethically interfere with an individual's choices when he or she cannot take these steps, or in a situation where the individual's chosen action interferes with the rights of others.

In the health care context, respect for autonomy means allowing and enabling patients to make their own choices. As therapists, our desire to help people sometimes causes us to show little respect for autonomy. Should patients choose not to participate in therapy, for example, our efforts to convince them otherwise shows our lack of respect for the patient's autonomy.

Nonmaleficence

Another ethical principle, nonmaleficence, embraces the message extrapolated from the Hippocratic Oath: "Do no harm" (Beauchamp & Childress, 1994). This principle, one of the oldest ethical principles, reminds us that if we cannot help patients, at the very least we have a duty not to harm them (Shannon, 1997). Harm encompasses a range of injuries extending beyond physical or psychological damage, including harm to one's reputation, liberty, or property. The questions of "Whose harm?" and "Which harms?" leave themselves open to many interpretations, especially when dealing with patients unable to make their own decisions.

Beneficence

A related ethical principle, beneficence, stands for the duty to prevent harm to others, to remove harm from others, and to promote good. One's obligation to this moral duty ends where action can bring harm to oneself. Often one must balance the duty to act with the harm acting may cause. For example, one has no moral duty to save a person from drowning if one cannot swim, although one has a duty to act, such as calling for help (Shannon, 1997). In the health care context, consider beneficence as looking out for the patient's well-being.

Justice

"Justice, sir, is the great interest of man on earth.
It is the ligament which holds civilized beings
and civilized nations together."
Daniel Webster, 1845

Justice considers ways of fairly distributing burdens and benefits in society and giving individuals their due. One can balance the needs of the individual with the needs of others in society competing for the same resources, which is called comparative justice. Alternatively, one can give each individual what he or she needs or wants, called noncomparative justice (Shannon, 1997). As more and more people compete for limited health care resources, the principle of justice takes a front seat in health care decision making.

OTHER ETHICAL TERMINOLOGY

Beyond the four basic ethical principles, readers will find that other ethical terms provide guidance in their analysis of ethical dilemmas. These terms give readers a basic vocabulary of ethics jargon.

Informed Consent

Informed consent obligates health care providers to present patients with the details, benefits, risks, and potential risks of all proposed intervention strategies, so patients can make willing, informed choices in their care. Obtaining informed consent relies heavily on another ethical principle—veracity.

Veracity

"I never did give anybody hell. I just told the truth
and they thought it was hell."
Harry S Truman, quoted in Baker, 1992

Veracity, one's obligation to speak and act truthfully, affects all communication with patients. For example, as previously discussed, informed consent requires disclosing certain information to the patient so the patient may make an informed choice. If the health care provider does not tell the truth, then the patient cannot make a truly informed decision. Therefore, one may only obtain informed consent based on truthful communication between the health care provider and the patient. As Harry S Truman reminds us, the truth sometimes hurts.

Confidentiality

Confidentiality—another essential term—also finds its roots in the Hippocratic Oath. The Hippocratic Oath, written in the fourth or fifth century BC and still affirmed by physicians today, states in part:

"Anything I see or hear of the life of men, whether
in a professional capacity or otherwise, which
should not be passed on to others, I will hold as
professional secrets and not divulge them."
Quoted in Hammonds v. Aetna Casualty & Surety Co., 243
F. Supp 793, 797 (N.D. Ohio 1965)

All health care providers have a duty or obligation to limit access to information gathered in the course of treatment and to keep the information strictly between the health care provider and the patient (Gert, Culver, & Clouser, 1997). Other ethical principles dictate some exceptions to the duty to keep patient information confidential. For example, based on principles of justice and beneficence, certain laws mandate breach of confidentiality to protect citizens, such as child abuse laws or other reporting laws designed to protect individuals who are mortally threatened.

Fidelity

Fidelity, a principle closely related to confidentiality, means the moral duty to keep promises and commitments (Beauchamp & Childress, 1994; Graber, 1998). Patients expect health care providers to keep their explicit and implicit promises, including the promise to keep shared information confidential (Beauchamp & Childress, 1994).

Duty

When we speak of duty, we refer to obligations individuals have to others in society. Sometimes those duties exist because of the nature of the relationship between the parties. For example, in the therapy arena, when we start a patient-therapist relationship, we have certain duties to the patient, such as a duty to provide a certain level of care and a duty of confidentiality.

Rights

Rights refer to the ability to take advantage of a moral entitlement to do something or not to do something. For example, in our society, individuals have a right to privacy and a right against self-incrimination. In an age of health care reform, many debate whether an individual has a right to health care or certain specified treatment.

Paternalism

Paternalism occurs when one fails to respect another's autonomy and acts with disregard to that individual's rights. When individuals act in a paternalistic manner, they substitute their beliefs, opin-ions, and judgments for the patient's judgment. Usually people justify paternalistic actions by claiming they acted in the person's best interest. This often occurs in health care.

PROFESSIONAL ETHICS

Health professionals deal with people fulfilling different roles: patients, family members, students, administrators, colleagues, support staff, and vendors. Each person comes to the relationship and situation with a different set of personal values, as well as professional values and religious and moral beliefs. Individuals involved in these relationships experience differences of opinion as well as conflicting goals and moral beliefs. Decision making involves making choices, and a person may reject values that differ from his or her own, or in a particular context, may have a conflict in his or her own values. Professional ethics incorporate those values, principles, and morals into professional decision making.

Professionals, dedicated to a common purpose and with common training, also draw from their training and professional obligations as another source of ethical values. Professional ethics and codes of professional ethics developed by professional associations enter the picture to guide the individual's behavior in circumscribed professional situations.

A professional code of ethics incorporates a set of rules or principles intended to express the particular values of the profession as a whole. Most professional codes of ethics consider ethical theory to some extent. Generally, professional associations develop professional codes of ethics through a process that includes input from the membership or organization's ethics committee, a peer review process, and a periodic review or update procedure. Once drafted and reviewed, professional codes of ethics often face a vote of the membership or a governing body of the association. One's membership in a professional association obligates the professional to abide by the association's code of ethics.

Often licensing boards and other credentialing agencies embrace and adopt or incorporate professional codes of ethics into their licensure regulations or credentialing rules. When this occurs, nonmembers of the professional association become subject to the profession's code of ethics even though they opt not to join the professional association.

Professional codes of ethics give meaning to many ethical terms and translate the terminology into concrete, understandable, practice-related language. Health and rehabilitation professionals should expect to find guidance and direction from professional codes of ethics. However, professional codes of ethics do not attempt to nor do they provide all of the answers to ethics questions. Sometimes, professional codes of ethics raise more questions for the professional or student who seeks definitive answers to ethical issues. One must realize codes of ethics often provide only a minimal standard for the profession.

Some professional codes of ethics provide more guidance than others. Some codes of ethics, such as those of the American Optometric Association (AOA) (1944), the American Pharmaceutical Association (1994), and the American Physical Therapy Association (APTA) (1991), consist of brief lists of key points. Other codes of ethics, such as those of the American Psychological Association (APA) (1992), the American College of Health Care Executives (ACHE) (1995), the American Occupational Therapy Association (AOTA) (1994), and the American Speech and Hearing Association (ASHA) (1994), provide more detailed and lengthy guidance.

Professional ethics in health care address several common themes and incorporate ethical principles. Health professionals often refer to themselves as "helping" professionals and therefore place professional value on beneficence or helping others. The theme of nonmaleficence, the directive to do no harm, relates closely to "helping."

Competency and confidentiality stand out as common subjects of professional codes of ethics in health care. Health and rehabilitation professionals find the autonomy of both the patient and the health care provider an important aspect of professional conduct in making decisions regarding treatment. The health professional's truthfulness or veracity in dealing with patients, families, other professionals, and health care providers defines another essential professional value. Finally, the requirement that one report the unethical behavior of others in the same profession remains a common theme among codes of ethics.

Rarely does a code of ethics provide a professional with an absolute guide to behavior or decision making in any given circumstance. The code of ethics provides a mere starting place or a point of reference to guide professional practice and decisions. The code of ethics exists as a set of values one must incorporate into a professional moral and behavioral repertoire in the same way an individual incorporates social, cultural, and religious values. The incorporation of social, cultural, and religious values occurs as a lifelong process during which many opportunities present themselves for trial and error learning, which for most individuals includes experiences with long-term teachers and role models.

Professional education, on the other hand, provides only a brief glimpse into the potential pitfalls of practice and little opportunity for the actual integration of professional values. Most professionals engage in on-the-job and by-the-seat-of-the-pants training, with little preparation for the application of a professional code of ethics to professional practice. Successful integration of ethical principles requires skill in the analysis of situations that arise in the current health care climate. As with the development of any skill, repetitive practice and opportunity for application of the skill play an essential role.

UNETHICAL PRACTICE

When one speaks of unethical practice, one refers to practice that does not conform to established professional standards. This includes practice that ranges from unreasonable, unjustified, and ineffective to immoral, questionable, and (knowingly) harmful or wrong. Every health professional can identify practices that he or she considers unethical. However, because we arrive at an ethical analysis from different social, religious, and cultural perspectives, not everyone will agree with our analysis. Whereas some may see a situation as a black and white issue, others may see variations of gray. An adage states that if you put two lawyers in a room, you end up with three different opinions. The same holds true when you put two health professionals together to review the same practice situation. More likely than not, they will reach at least three conclusions as to which action or actions fall under the umbrella of ethical practice.

Unethical practice affects the patient, the health

care professional, the organization, insurance providers, and society. Unethical practice can cause serious individual consequences with potentially far-reaching social ramifications.

For example, newspaper headlines contain widely publicized instances of health professionals who, because of their dedication to relieving human suffering, acted on their perceived role and withdrew life support or administered lethal doses of medication. The consequence to the individual professional is long-term incarceration for committing a crime. The consequence to the patient is death. The social ramification could be universal mistrust of health professionals, resulting in underutilization of services and increased health problems. The consequences of unethical practice vary, as do the perceptions of what is unethical, the situations in which the unethical behavior occurs, and the range of society's response, varying from incarceration to simply ignoring or even condoning unethical behavior.

SUMMARY

Ethical theories and concepts together with professional codes of ethics provide a foundation for understanding one's responsibilities in terms of ethical decision making. Personal and professional ethics play a role in one's concepts of ethical and unethical behavior within a professional context.

REFERENCES

American College of Health Care Executives (1995). *Code of ethics*. Available http://www.ache.org/code.html.

American Occupational Therapy Association (1994). *Occupational therapy code of ethics*. Available http://www.aota.org/aotaarea/frameeth.html.

American Optometric Association (1944). *Code of ethics*. Center for the Study of Ethics in the Professions, Illinois Institute of Technology. Available http://csep.iit.edu/codes/coe/aopt-a.htm.

American Pharmaceutical Association (1994). *The study of ethics in the professions*. Illinois Institute of Technology. Available http://csep.iit.edu/codes/coe/American%20Phamceutical%20Association%20Code%20of%20Ethics_2.html.

American Physical Therapy Association (1991). *Code of ethics*. Available http://www.apta.org/Ethics/code_of_ethics.html.

American Psychological Association (1992). *Center for the study of ethics in the professions*. Illinois Institute of Technology. Available http://csep.iit.edu/codes/coe/apsych-u.htm.

American Speech and Hearing Association (1994). *Code of ethics*. Available http://www.asha.org/professionals/library/code_of_ethics.htm].

Arras, J. D. (1998). Getting down to cases: The revival of casuistry in bioethics. In J. F. Monagle & D. C. Thomasma. (Eds.). *Health care ethics*. Gaithersburg, MD: Aspen.

Baker, D. B. (1992). *Power quotes*. Detroit, MI: Visible Ink Press.

Beauchamp, T. L., & Childress, J. F. (1994). *Principles of biomedical ethics*. New York: Oxford University Press.

Gardner, J. W., & Reese, F. G. (1996). *Wit & wisdom*. New York: W.W. Norton & Company.

Gert, B., Culver, C. M., & Clouser K. D. (1997). *Bioethics: A return to fundamentals*. New York: Oxford University Press.

Graber, G. C. (1998). Basic theories in medical ethics. In J. F. Monagle & D. C. Thomasma. (Eds.). *Health care ethics*. Gaithersburg, MD: Aspen.

Hammonds v. Aetna Casualty & Surety Co. 243 F. Supp 793 (N.D. Ohio 1965).

Jonsen, Seigler, & Winslade (1998). *Clinical ethics*. New York: McGraw Hill.

Monagle, J. F. (1998). Ethical responsible creativity. In J. F. Monagle & D. C. Thomasma (Eds.). *Health care ethics*. Gaithersburg, MD: Aspen.

Peter, L. J. (1977). *Peter's quotations*. New York: Quill, William Morrow.

Shannon, T. A. (1997). *An introduction to bioethics*. New York: Paulist Press.

Sim, J. (1997). *Ethical decision making in practice*. Oxford, UK: Butterworth Heinemann.

3

Legal Issues in Ethical Decision Making

"Morality cannot be legislated, but behavior can be regulated. Judicial decrees may not change the heart, but they can restrain the heartless."

Martin Luther King, Jr., quoted in Baker, 1992

Practicing in the health care arena at the dawn of the millennium is complicated. Ever-changing laws and regulations change the way therapy practitioners conduct their business. The changing laws and regulations raise numerous legal issues that therapy practitioners cannot avoid, especially while trying to maintain one's practice within ethical standards.

Numerous legal issues affect ethical decision making in practice. Often, when faced with an ethical dilemma, a legal issue looms in the background. For example, in analyzing a reimbursement issue, readers should question whether a proposed alternative action violates Medicare laws or regulations. A dilemma concerning the alternatives a pediatric practitioner should consider if he or she suspects child abuse should make one question whether state law requires the therapist to report suspected child abuse. Many scenarios raise legal red flags.

This chapter examines some of the more common legal issues therapists may face in dealing with today's ethical dilemmas and provides "how to's" to avoid or minimize problems with these legal issues. The authors do not expect therapy practitioners to become attorneys, but readers should acquire some familiarity with legal issues affecting ethical decision making. Readers will find many of the references cited here excerpted in the appendices to assist with the ethical dilemma analysis process. Internet

references refer readers to others. Before getting into specifics of law, readers should understand some basic principles.

This chapter addresses statutory laws—both federal and state. Federal laws are passed by Congress in Washington, DC, and apply to all 50 states and territories of the United States. Examples of federal laws include copyright laws, IDEA (Individuals with Disabilities Education Act), antitrust laws, and Medicare laws. Federal copyright laws, for example, apply anywhere in the United States.

Certain laws fall under the umbrella of state law. State legislatures vote to enact state laws, so unlike federal laws, state laws may vary from state to state. Whereas the sample laws excerpted in the appendices will help readers complete some of the practice exercises in this workbook, readers' state laws will probably vary from those found in this text. Readers may also find themes common to both the excerpted laws in the appendices and those in their own state, whereas others appear to vary greatly. For example, some state statutes include elder abuse laws; others do not. Therefore, this chapter addresses general state themes. Readers may need to fill in specifics with information about laws from their own states, which may or may not prescribe certain responsibilities on therapy practitioners. Readers will find the internet a good starting point for locating state laws.

Both state and federal laws change over time as legislative bodies pass new laws. A legislative body may amend or repeal a law imposing additional responsibilities on the practitioner. Despite this imposition of additional legal responsibility, the law may not impose a requirement that the government actually notify individuals of these changes on an individual basis. In other words, the government will probably not send you a letter notifying you of a new legal requirement to do something under penalty of fine, imprisonment, or loss of license. The law assumes you have notice of the change once the notice appears in a government document, such as the *Federal Registry* or its equivalent state-level publication. The legal system refers to this as "record notice." Record notice imposes a responsibility on the individual to make himself or herself aware of new laws as they take effect.

National professional associations provide a good service of notifying their members of these changes when the change involves a federal law. State professional associations often publish changes in their newsletter when the changes involve state laws. Licensure boards, such as those in Florida and Georgia, often send newsletters informing licensees of new requirements imposed under the licensure law or regulations.

In addition to requirements imposed by laws (also called statutes) themselves, readers face requirements imposed by regulations. Both federal and state laws carry with them regulations. Regulations, promulgated by administrative bodies such as licensure boards (state) or the Health Care Finance Administration (HCFA) (federal) with input from the public, provide more specific information or blueprints exacting how the fine points of the law will play out in the real world. For example, a licensure law may require continuing education and may prescribe the number of continuing education credits one must take. The regulations promulgated by the licensure board will specify the procedures for reporting continuing education credits and how providers of continuing education meet the certification requirements. Similarly, on a federal level, Medicare law mandates the provision of certain services, whereas the Medicare regulations define who may provide those services. Thus, in analyzing an ethical dilemma, an issue might arise in which the therapist finds guidance from both a law and a regu-

lation. Readers may access many regulations on the Internet.

Laws fall into one of two categories: criminal or civil. A criminal law imposes criminal penalties such as a fine, imprisonment, or forfeiture of property for violations of either state or federal criminal laws— referred to as a crime against the state. Should an individual murder another, the state will prosecute the alleged murderer under a criminal statute. Civil matters infringe on the rights of an individual, which can also include a company or employer. For example, in the infamous O.J. Simpson case, the victim's father, Fred Goldman, sued O.J. Simpson in civil court, alleging that Mr. Simpson infringed on his rights by depriving him of his son.

In addition to statutory law, the body of law in the United States also includes judge-made law, also called "common law." As part of the decision-making process that comes before the courts, judges analyze statutes, interpret them, and apply them to the facts of specific cases before them, thereby creating common law, sometimes called "case law."

Obviously, this book cannot address every possible legal issue that might arise in the course of analyzing ethical dilemmas. However, a discussion of legal issues is not complete without some mention of the relationship between legal and ethical conduct. Therefore, the authors provide a look at potential legal issues more common to the dilemmas provided in the workbook portion of this book. Readers must consider legal issues together with ethical issues. For additional information about specific legal issues, readers may want to consult an attorney (Figure 3-1).

In addition to the legal considerations that govern the professional conduct of therapists, professional codes of ethics also guide the conduct of therapists. (See Appendix A for sample codes of ethics.) Professional ethical standards tend to cover areas of practice deemed undesirable or unacceptable by the profession, although not expressly prohibited by law.

"In a civilized life, law floats in a sea of ethics."
Justice Earl Warren, 1962, quoted in Baker, 1992

In some situations, courts will look at the ethical standards of a profession. Without any clear legal authority governing the conduct of a therapy practitioner, the courts may need to find a standard of care to govern the occupational therapy consultant's conduct. The courts may look to the standard of care of a similarly situated professional, or the court may look to the profession's self-imposed standards to determine potential liability (Hertfelder & Crispen, 1990).

Although no court has yet interpreted the Occupational Therapy Code of Ethics, for example, as a basis for determining the conduct of an occupational therapist, the possibility remains for its future use by a court of law. Courts have already interpreted ethical guidelines and standards of care belonging to the medical, legal, and accounting professions. It is likely that the courts would do the same with the occupational, physical therapy, and speech pathology codes of ethics and standards of practice, should the situation arise. Thus, therapy practitioners could protect themselves from potential legal liability by following the code of ethics and standards of practice promulgated by their profession.

LICENSURE

Licensure provides another standard of conduct for therapy practitioners. As previously mentioned, states control licensure through state laws and regulations. Therefore, requirements for licensure vary from state to state. One must understand the rudiments of licensure to practice within legal, as well as ethical, parameters (see Appendix B).

States enact licensure laws to protect the public. To meet this purpose, licensure laws usually prescribe the type of behavior therapists must follow within the state, often incorporating the professional association's code of ethics.

The licensure laws also list penalties for those who participate in the behaviors they prohibit. Licensure laws refer to the process of assigning penalties for unacceptable behaviors as "disciplinary action." Violating the state's licensure law subjects one to the disciplinary process. The penalties one may face through disciplinary action may range from fines to suspension or revocation of one's license. Although the specific, enumerated prohibited behaviors vary from state to state, some behaviors that typically subject licensed practitioners to disciplinary action under licensure laws include engaging in sexual relations with a patient, accepting kickbacks, promoting the practice of the profession by unlicensed persons, and otherwise taking advantage of

patients. See Table 3-1 for additional behaviors that may subject one to disciplinary action.

Every practitioner should read his or her licensure law (often called a "practice act") to determine which behaviors his or her state specifically prohibits. Licensure laws contain information readers will find invaluable in solving many ethical dilemmas. After reading one's practice act, an ethical dilemma may transform into an obvious choice rather than a dilemma. Reviewing the licensure law can answer many questions and familiarity with the practice act can keep practitioners out of trouble.

In addition to the licensure law, practitioners should read the law's implementing regulations. In most cases, the licensure board promulgates the regulations, which may include continuing education requirements, disciplinary procedures, supervision requirements, and the specific steps one must take to acquire a license. Knowledge of these regulations also provides readers with important information for solving ethical dilemmas. Staying on top of the regulations and changes as they occur can also help keep practitioners from losing their licenses.

CHILD, SPOUSE, AND ELDER ABUSE

In addition to licensure, other laws impose legal duties and obligations on therapy practitioners. One might see these obligations assessed with child, spouse, and elder abuse. In an effort to protect their citizens, many states go beyond prohibiting child, spouse, and elder abuse. These states require certain professionals to report suspected abuse. Some states require health professionals to report suspected child abuse only, whereas others include spouse and elder abuse as well. Some states require only that physicians report suspected abuse whereas others extend this requirement to other professionals, such as all health professionals, teachers, and day care workers. The state's legal requirement to report abuse serves as an exception to the patient confidentiality requirement of licensure laws.

Readers may find their role as therapist obligates them to report abuse according to the state law requirement (see Appendix E). Many states put in place abuse hotlines to allow those who report abuse to remain anonymous. Ethical dilemmas may arise when therapists find the legal obligation to report

Table 3-1

Behaviors That May Subject Licensees to Disciplinary Action

- ◆ Abuse of drugs or alcohol
- ◆ Conviction of a felony
- ◆ Conviction of a crime of moral turpitude
- ◆ Conviction of a crime related to the practice of the profession for which one holds a license
- ◆ Practicing without a prescription or referral (if required by the state's practice act)
- ◆ Applying electrical modalities without proper training (for occupational therapy in some states)
- ◆ Obtaining a license using fraud or deception
- ◆ Gross negligence in practicing one's profession
- ◆ Breaching patient confidentiality
- ◆ Failing to report a known violation of the licensure law by another licensee
- ◆ Making or filing false claims or reports
- ◆ Accepting kickbacks
- ◆ Deceptive advertising
- ◆ Exercising undue influence over patients or clients
- ◆ Failing to maintain adequate records
- ◆ Failing to provide adequate supervision
- ◆ Providing unnecessary services
- ◆ False, deceptive, or misleading advertising
- ◆ Practicing under a name other than one's own
- ◆ Failure to perform a legal obligation
- ◆ Practicing medicine
- ◆ Performing services not authorized by the patient
- ◆ Performing experimental services without first obtaining informed consent
- ◆ Practicing beyond scope permitted
- ◆ Failing to comply with continuing education requirements
- ◆ Inability to practice competently
- ◆ Engaging in sexual relations with a patient

abuse in conflict with the employing facility's policies and procedures.

CONTRACTS

"A verbal contract isn't worth the paper it's written on."
Samuel Goldwyn, quoted in Peter, 1977

Legal and ethical issues often arise surrounding the complexities and intricacies of contracts. When two parties make an agreement with mutual promises, they form a contract. As health professionals, therapists work in many situations where they may encounter contractual relationships. For example, therapists enter into contracts with their employers, commonly referred to as employment contracts. Therapists may also find themselves involved in contractual relationships with managed care companies or other providers or insurers to provide therapy services.

As part of the contract, the parties agree to specific terms. For example, a therapist might agree to work in exchange for a set amount of wages and benefits. By signing the contract, parties (employer and employee) bind themselves to follow the specific terms outlined in the contract. As another example, in a contract between a hospital or therapist in private practice and a health maintenance organization (HMO), one might find a gag clause restricting the range of information a therapist may discuss with patients (Martin & Bjerknes, 1996).

Noncompete Clauses

Therapists may also encounter noncompete clauses as terms in employment contracts. This term restricts the therapist from working in a particular geographic location for a particular period of time following the termination of the contract. For example, a simple noncompete clause might read as follows:

The therapist agrees not to work for any nursing homes or rehabilitation clinics within a 10-mile radius of the Shady Rest Nursing Home for a period of 2 years from the time s/he leaves employment with the Company.

More detailed noncompete clauses, in addition to the above, may add something like the following:

The therapist agrees not to solicit, directly or indirectly, any patients or clients of the Company or interfere in any way with the Company's relationships with any facility with which it has an established contractual relationship.

Parties to contracts may need to seek assistance of the courts to enforce or contest a noncompete clause. Courts usually uphold noncompete clauses where they find the clauses reasonable in time—meaning duration—and distance-meaning geographic area covered (Stromberg, et al., 1988).

Breach of Contract

When a party to a contract fails to live up to his or her end of the contractual agreement, we say that party breached the contract. For example, suppose a therapist signs a contract containing a noncompete clause agreeing not to work directly for the nursing home with which the rehabilitation company contracts. Following her resignation, the therapist takes a job working for the nursing home where she previously worked under contract with a rehabilitation company. By taking a job working directly for the nursing home, the therapist breaches the contract. As a civil matter, this breach of contract places the therapist in a position to pay damages should the rehabilitation company choose to sue her.

In contracts with noncompete clauses, employers often include in the contract the damages they may seek and the allocation or computation of those damages should the therapist breech the contract by violating the noncompete clause. For example, the employer might seek an injunction against the therapist and seek from the therapist the costs incurred in suing. The contract may also include a specific monetary amount as damages in case the therapist should violate the noncompete clause.

In addition to the legal implications, breach of contract often raises ethical concerns as well; for example, when in breaching their contracts therapists abandon patients, fail to complete their documentation on time, or "borrow" (either permanently or temporarily) company records including patient charts.

Confidentiality Clauses and Trade Secrets

Some contracts include clauses requiring that the therapist not disclose certain proprietary information which, if disclosed to competitors, could cause the employer detrimental results. This proprietary information often carries the label "trade secrets." A trade secret refers to a "formula, pattern, device, or information that is used in the operation of a business and provides the business an advantage or an opportunity to obtain an advantage over those who do not know or use it" (Fla Stat § 812.081). Trade secrets include information "including a formula, pattern, compilation, program, device, or process ..." (Fla Stat §688.002[4]). In the technical world, the concept of trade secrets covers items such as computer programs, product design plans, and chemical formulas. For example, imagine what would happen if an employee of Coca-Cola gave its formula, a trade secret, to one of Coca-Cola's competitors.

The therapy world shares this concern with Coca-Cola. In the therapy context, the proprietary information might include billing systems, forms, training manuals, home program materials, referral source lists, patient lists, charge masters, HMO contracts, or information regarding allegations of malpractice. This prohibition against disclosure continues to bind the therapist after he or she leaves the employer.

Sometimes employers include a penalty in the contract, which it may enforce through the courts should therapists violate the confidentiality clause. As with the nondisclosure clauses, penalties may include money damages, issuance of an injunction, or other relief. Therapists who use another's proprietary information may also find themselves facing allegations of theft, also called misappropriation of a trade secret (Fla Stat §688.003[1]; *Board of Regents v. Taborsky*, 648 So. 2d 748 [Fla. 2d DCA 1994]).

Therapists should read any contracts before they

sign them. Therapists should make sure they understand the terms of the contract before signing them and review with an attorney any confusing or unclear clauses they may find before signing the contract. Above all, therapists should keep a copy of the contract for their records.

Work for Hire and Copyright

Ownership of materials one creates for one's employer and ideas one puts to paper while in someone's employ often raise legal and ethical issues for therapy practitioners. Employers often ask therapists to create written materials for them as part of their job responsibilities. In the therapy arena, this might include, for example, home program worksheets, evaluation forms, and family/caregiver training materials. Once a therapist creates these materials for the employer, they become the employer's proprietary interest. Put simply, work created for an employer belongs to the employer. We call these documents "work for hire" (Stromberg, et al., 1988). Therapists cannot copyright these materials in their own names. After therapists leave the job with the employer, they may not take the items with them to use with another employer. If one does, one may commit a copyright violation or face a charge of theft of company secrets.

Independent Contractor Relationship

Another hot topic in the therapy community that raises ethical and legal eyebrows concerns the issue of whether an individual belongs in the employee or independent contractor category. The authors of this book repeatedly encounter therapy professionals who erroneously refer to themselves as "independent contractors." The therapy professional subscribes to the notion that because one is self-employed, employed part-time, or paid on an hourly basis, he or she qualifies as an independent contractor. Therapy professionals must familiarize themselves with the dangers of erroneously classifying an employee as an independent contractor. A misclassification of an employee as an independent contractor can cost the employer back taxes plus penalties. Depending on one's state laws, employers will also find themselves facing additional penalties should a workers' compensation injury occur to an independent contractor whom courts deem an employee.

The law bases the relationship between an employer and employees on a contract. The terms *employer* and *employee* come from the common law terminology *master and servant*. Master and servant indicates a relationship exists in which one person who employs another has control over the manner in which he or she performs the work. The employer is the master over the work of the servant, or employee (Makar, 1996).

An employer can tell the employee precisely how he or she wants the job done. The employer can tell the employee what time to report to work, how to perform the job, when to perform the job, and to what standards. An employer may also terminate the employee if he or she fails to perform according to the employer's standards.

Not all therapy professionals who provide therapy services will fit squarely in the employee category. One can structure a relationship with a therapy professional so he or she may qualify as an independent contractor. The independent contractor relationship finds its roots in the contractual relationship with another person or entity to perform a task. However, persons seeking the services of independent contractors cannot control their performance and must concern themselves only with the results. The difference between the employer-employee relationship and the employer-independent contractor relationship depends mostly on the right of control over the work (1 Restatement of Law, Agency [2nd ed.] § 220 [2] 1957). Remember, under the law, the therapy professional in the independent contractor relationship is a private practitioner.

The mere existence of a written contract agreeing to the independent contractor status and the absence of withholding taxes does not make one an independent contractor. Home health agencies sometimes hire therapy professionals to provide direct therapy in home health care. The agencies call these therapists independent contractors merely because they sign a contract and agree to accept payment on a per-treatment basis, without any payroll taxes withheld or social security taxes or worker's compensation insurance paid by the agency. These home health agencies and nursing services have come under very strict scrutiny from the Internal Revenue Service (IRS) (Weinstein, 1991).

The authors have often heard therapy professionals comment that an individual is "just an independent contractor" when referring to a part-time employee. One does not become an independent contractor by agreement between the prospective employer and a potential "therapist-for-hire." One does not become an independent contractor by designation by the employer. While it may sound like a simple way to avoid the administrative headaches of paying payroll, benefits, and social security taxes, designating an employee as an independent contractor can bring painful consequences.

Before signing contracts, employers should make sure therapy professionals meet the criteria for an independent contractor. Both the IRS and common law use specific tests for making this determination. The tests involve reviewing a set of factors to determine whether the employer accurately designated an individual as an independent contractor.

The common law test, developed from decisions of previous appellate court cases, gives the court guidance should a question arise about workers' compensation. The court's goal in the common law test is to determine whether the employer has the legal right to control both the method and result of the services.

To answer this question, the common law has developed a test that includes 10 factors (see Appendix K). The courts will look at each factor and apply the facts of the particular case to the individual factors.

The IRS guidelines consist of a similar inquiry to determine the accuracy of a worker's status as employee or independent contractor. The IRS looks at whether the person or persons for whom the services are performed exercise sufficient control over the individual for the individual to fall into the employee category (Rev. Rul. 87-41, CB 1987-1, 296). This inquiry involves 20 factors set forth by the IRS (Weinstein, 1991) (see Appendix C).

Problems arise in the therapy arena when two therapy professionals work side-by-side performing identical jobs, but one holds the title "employee" while the other holds the title "independent contractor." Therapy professionals confused with their status might want to contact an attorney for advice and guidance.

Those therapy professionals wishing to maintain an independent contractor status may take steps to preserve their independence. Independent contractors should perform services pursuant to written contracts for a stipulated period of time, not terminable at will. The parties must follow the terms of the contract.

The contract should refrain from any mention of control by the person or entity contracting for the services. For example, one would not want to include a control provision specifying the independent contractor must follow all policies of the employer in an independent contractor agreement.

Beware if you see the words "employment contract" across the top of the contract. The authors have seen this phrase in independent contractor contracts with home health agencies. As a general rule, never use the words "employee" or "employer" in a contract with an independent contractor. In the contract, always refer to the independent contractor as the "independent contractor," "therapist," or "therapy professional." The contracting party should resist the temptation to refer to itself as the "employer." Rather, in the contract with the independent contractor, use the term "company," "corporation," or the name of the company.

The contract should also allow the worker to reject jobs offered to him or her without penalty. The worker must also retain the right, under the terms of the contract, to select other employment opportunities.

FRAUD

Fraud, another issue overshadowing therapy practice today, raises legal and ethical red flags. Fraud occurs when an individual makes misrepresentations or lies in order to induce an entity or an individual to do something or refrain from doing something (Darken, 1997). In the therapy context, fraud often occurs in the context of billing. Common misrepresentations in the therapy world include billing for services never provided, billing for more services than were actually provided, or billing non-covered services as covered services.

For example, in many parts of the country, Blue Cross does not cover outpatient occupational therapy services. Suppose a physician refers a patient to outpatient occupational therapy services for hand therapy. If the occupational therapist were to treat the patient, and the facility billed the treatment as physical therapy so it could receive payment, the facility would commit insurance fraud, which is now a federal crime (Darken, 1997) (see Appendices D and I). Further, should therapists submit their fraudulent billings or other documentation through the mail, they may find themselves facing federal criminal charges of mail fraud (see Appendices D and I). Federal law also provides for a separate criminal charge should the therapists submit fraudulent materials electronically over telephone wire (Health Care Portability and Accountability Act of 1996, Public Law 104-191 [1996]; Darken, 1997).

Other fraudulent practices include backdating notes and fabricating notes for visits never made. Readers will find many examples of fraudulent billing practices in the ethical dilemmas in this book.

Medicare Fraud

Unfortunately, Medicare fraud in the provision of therapy services receives much national media attention and flirts with therapy professionals both legally and ethically. Medicare fraud occurs when a provider of therapy services knowingly or willingly lies to get paid (see Appendix M). Medicare abuse occurs whenever Medicare pays for an item or service it should not or anytime a provider bills Medicare for services not medically necessary (see Appendices M, D, and I) (Darken, 1997; MacDonald, Meyer, & Essig, 1985; Rosenblatt, Law, & Rosenbaum, 1997). For example, Medicare does not reimburse individually for therapeutic recreation visits. It does, however, pay for occupational therapy, physical therapy, and speech pathology services. If a facility bills therapeutic recreation services as occupational therapy, the facility commits fraud. Many practice acts and codes of ethics require therapists to report illegal activities such as these. If one fails to report illegal activity (Table 3-2), in addition to violating one's professional code of ethics and practice act, one may face federal criminal charges of conspiracy to cover up the Medicare fraud.

CONSPIRACY

Efforts to cover up Medicare fraud can unknowingly, or unwillingly, raise conspiracy issues for therapy professionals. A conspiracy occurs when individuals work together to commit a crime or to cover up evidence of the crime. Under the law, conspiracy constitutes a separate crime from the crime about which individuals conspire.

In the example from the previous section, suppose the facility were billing therapeutic recreation as occupational therapy, and the therapists knew the facility billed therapeutic recreation as occupational therapy. If the facility continued to submit the incorrect or fraudulent billing and the occupational therapists cosigned the therapeutic recreation notes knowing they were not occupational therapy notes, the therapists could find themselves charged with, among other things, conspiracy to commit Medicare fraud. Congress made clear the conspiracy law extended to the "ostrich with its head in the sand," when government contractors claimed no personal knowledge that overcharges occurred (Salcido, 1996). The therapists need not even know the billing scheme is illegal to face these charges.

In these days of managed care and health care reform, supervisors may instruct therapists to partake in activities outside the therapist's comfort zone. Perhaps the therapist questions whether the activity passes legal or ethical muster. To protect oneself from committing fraudulent activities and participating in conspiracies to commit fraud, therapists should ask for written instructions for these questionable activities or copies of written policies explaining what the therapist considers a questionable practice. Most people will not put illegal or unethical practices in writing.

MALPRACTICE

Malpractice raises many legal and ethical issues for therapy practitioners. Most claims of malpractice rest their contentions on the theory of negligence. Negligence occurs when the therapist's conduct falls below the acceptable standard of care for the profession. The therapist need not intend to do something poorly. Negligence concerns itself with one's conduct, not one's state of mind.

To prove malpractice under a theory of negligence, one must prove four elements:
1. A duty to act in a particular way
2. Conduct that breaches that duty
3. Damages
4. Conduct that falls below the standard of care, causing injury to the patient or client

First, a relationship between the parties must

Table 3-2
Acts Prohibited By Medicare and Medicare Fraud and Abuse Provisions* ◆ Making false claims for payment ◆ Making false statements for payment ◆ Billing for visits never made ◆ Billing for nonface-to-face therapy services ◆ Paying or receiving kickbacks for goods and services ◆ Soliciting for, making an offer for payment, paying, or receiving payment for patient referrals

*According to the HCFA

exist that creates a duty to act in a particular way. Second, the plaintiff must prove the therapy professional's conduct fell below the professionally reasonable standard of care, thereby breaching that duty to act in a particular way. Third, the plaintiff must prove he or she suffered real damages. Finally, the plaintiff must prove the therapy professional's breech of duty actually caused the damages suffered (Calloway, 1985; Hoffman, 1995; Makar, 1996; Prosser, 1971; Ranke & Moriarty, 1997).

A Duty to Act in a Particular Way

The therapy professional owes a duty to those patients or clients with whom he or she establishes a relationship. Thus, the therapy professional owes a duty of care to his or her patients and clients (Prosser, 1971). The duty owed applies to acts of omission and acts of commission. This means that therapy professionals can find themselves liable for damages caused by things they did, as well as things they failed to do (Makar, 1996).

The therapy professional's duty compels him or her to exercise the reasonable care and skills expected of a reasonably prudent therapy practitioner. The courts will inquire as to whether a reasonably prudent therapy practitioner would have acted in a similar manner given the same set of circumstances (Ranke & Moriarty, 1997).

Breach of Duty

The second element of malpractice, breach of duty, occurs when the therapy practitioner's conduct falls below the applicable standard of care. Expert witness testimony will help form the basis of proof at

trial for the standard of care. The expert witness, another therapy practitioner in the same field, will testify as to his or her opinion of the standard up to which the therapy practitioner's conduct should have measured (Ranke & Moriarty, 1997). Courts also may find themselves interpreting professional codes of ethics for assistance in establishing the standard of care.

Under the doctrine of *respondent superior*, the therapy practitioner may find himself or herself liable for actions of subordinates. This Latin term means "let the master answer" (Maker, 1996). Because the employer occupies the best position to supervise and direct acts of his or her employees within the scope of his or her employment, the law imputes liability to the employer under this doctrine. Because the basis for this doctrine comes from the right of control, the doctrine of respondent superior does not apply to independent contractors (Calloway, 1985; Ranke & Moriarty, 1997).

The therapy practitioner may find himself or herself liable for the actions of subordinates under another theory. Therapy practitioners may find themselves liable for negligent supervision if, for example, they assign others to perform therapy services they lack the qualification to perform and then fail to supervise them properly (Hopkins & Anderson, 1990; Stromberg et al., 1988).

Damages

One must prove this third element to sustain an action for malpractice, damages, or actual harm (Prosser, 1971). Harm caused by the therapy practitioner may include, for example, a plethora of physical harms to a patient/client. Even if the therapy practitioner acts in a clearly incompetent manner, no basis for a malpractice action exists absent proof of actual harm (Calloway, 1985).

On the other hand, if the therapy practitioner acts in a reasonable manner and provides appropriate therapeutic interventions, but the patient's condition does not improve, this harm alone does not constitute malpractice.

Causation of Injury to the Patient

Causation remains as the fourth element required to sustain a cause of action for malpractice. The plaintiff must show the therapy practitioner's negligent conduct was responsible for the plaintiff's injury. The standard is the "but for" test. In other words, but for the therapy practitioner's negligence, the plaintiff's injury would not have occurred.

ASSAULT AND BATTERY

Because therapy practitioners often come into physical contact with patients and clients, they need to familiarize themselves with legal and ethical issues involved with assault and battery issues. Although readers may already know about assault and battery in the criminal context, these terms also describe a civil act called a *tort*. Whereas malpractice is an unintentional act, assault and battery fall under the umbrella of intentional act called *intentional torts* (Hoffman, 1995). Assault occurs when someone commits an act that puts another individual in apprehension of being touched in an offensive manner (*Blacks*, 1979). In other words, someone puts the individual in apprehension of immediate bodily harm without consent. One need not actually touch the individual. Rather, the threat of harm meets the criteria.

Battery occurs when someone intentionally touches an individual without consent (Hoffman, 1995). The law recognizes that an individual has the right to freedom from invasion of his or her person. When an assault or battery occurs, the law recognizes the invasion of the individual's right to freedom from invasion of his or her person and provides the injured person with damages as a remedy for that invasion. Questions of assault and battery may arise in practice where, for example, someone puts an individual in restraints without doctor's orders.

INFORMED CONSENT

Most states today treat failure to obtain informed consent prior to treating a patient as a negligent act rather than an intentional tort, such as assault and battery. Thus, therapists may find themselves "negligent" should they treat a patient without first obtaining informed consent from the patient or client. Regardless of what the law says, codes of ethics and most licensure laws require practitioners to obtain informed consent prior to treatment. Licensure laws, codes of ethics, and a plethora of federal and state laws and regulations also require practitioners to obtain informed consent before including patients as subjects in research (Areen, King, Goldberg, Gostin, & Capron, 1996) (see 45 CFR 46 [1994]).

To obtain informed consent for treatment, practitioners must meet three requirements:

1. The practitioner must assure that the patient understands the procedure or treatment, its risks, potential benefits, and any available alternatives;
2. The patient must freely give consent, meaning willingly and without duress; and
3. The patient must possess the capacity to legally give consent (Biano & Hirsh, 1995).

One problem therapists may face with informed consent arises if they contract with managed care companies. Suppose the managed care company imposes a gag rule as a term in its contractual agreement with the therapist. A case manager in the managed care company authorizes a particular treatment and only that treatment. Common sense tells the therapist that once the case manager makes a decision, the patient has no choice in making treatment decisions. Further, facing a gag rule, the therapist may find himself or herself unable to present patients with treatment alternatives and other necessary information, thereby making it impossible to obtain informed consent from the patient (Martin & Bjerknes, 1996).

Other situations exist where therapists may also find obtaining informed consent difficult. Often, therapists find their patients or clients unable to give informed consent for a variety of reasons. For example, a patient declared incompetent cannot give informed consent. A parent or guardian must give informed consent for a child. Sometimes patients lack the ability to give informed consent because their medical condition interferes with their ability to understand or ask questions about the informed consent process. Further, a patient who does not wish to participate in therapy will refuse to give informed consent.

GUARDIANSHIP/CONSERVATORSHIP

When the state finds an individual cannot care for his or her needs, because of age in the case of children or incompetence in the case of adults, the state appoints a guardian to take care of the individual's needs. This may occur with patients following traumatic brain injury or the onset of Alzheimer's disease, for example. Some states refer to the guardian as a *conservator*. The legal system refers to the incapacitated individual or child as the *ward*.

Therapists need to understand this relationship because therapists often find themselves working with patients in the care of the guardian. When the state appoints a guardian, the ward loses all or some of his or her rights, the scope of which depends on the state. For example, in most cases, when under a guardian's care, a patient lacks the capacity to give consent for treatment. All authorization for treatment as well as payment must come from the guardian or conservator. The ward cannot give informed consent.

Often, states appoint family members as guardians. These same guardians often are the heirs of the estate of the ward. Thus, the guardian may not find it in his or her interest to spend the ward's money on therapy. This can present ethical as well legal dilemmas for therapists.

ANTITRUST

Changes in the health care system bring antitrust issues to the forefront for therapy professionals. In *Northern Pacific Railway v. United States*, 365 U.S. 1, 4-5 (1958), the United States Supreme Court explained the purpose of the U.S. antitrust laws:

The Sherman (Antitrust) Act was designed to be a comprehensive charter of economic liberty aimed at preserving free and unfettered competition as the rule of trade. It rests on the premise that unrestrained interaction of competitive forces will yield the best allocation of our economic resources, the lowest prices, the highest quality, and the greatest material progress.

Antitrust laws seek to prohibit practices that interfere with this free competition.

Typical practices violating antitrust laws include price fixing, division of markets, and boycotts. The Supreme Court applied the antitrust law to health care in the case of *Arizona v. Maricopa County Medical Society*, 457 U.S. 332 (1982). In Maricopa, physicians in the medical society agreed to set a maximum fee for their services. The court found setting maximum fees was illegal price fixing and in violation of antitrust laws.

The decision in the Maricopa case suggests therapists avoid discussing fees when they gather in professional groups. Readers will find antitrust issues hot topics in the near future and ripe for modification as managed care's hold tightens. Much of managed care contracting rests on setting fees. In many locations, therapists' responses to managed care's stronghold include forming networks, which also involves agreements as to fees.

Other flirtations with antitrust in the current market include the merger and acquisition of numerous hospitals and clinics, leaving individual markets controlled by a small number of rather large health care corporations (Greaney, 1997).

EMBEZZLEMENT AND THEFT

Embezzlement occurs when an individual willfully takes someone else's property or money and uses it for his or her own (Blacks, 1978). Some sort of relationship must exist between the parties, such as an employer-employee relationship.

Theft occurs when an individual takes someone else's property without the owner's consent (Blacks, 1978). Unlike embezzlement, no relationship need exist between the parties.

Those who partake in embezzlement, theft, or both face criminal penalties if caught. Theft and embezzlement arise in the therapy context in several ways. First, section 243 of the Health Care Portability and Accountability Act of 1996, Public Law 104-191, created a new crime of theft and embezzlement. According to this law, one could spend a maximum of 10 years in prison for knowingly and willfully embezzling, stealing, intentionally misapplying, or otherwise taking for one's own use money, property, or other assets of a health care program that exceeded $100 in value (Health Care Portability Act, § 243; Darken, 1997).

Another type of embezzlement occurs when therapy practitioners permanently "borrow" items from their employers. Embezzlement and theft can also occur when therapy practitioners ask for reimbursement for items from "petty cash" that they did not purchase for the facility, or exaggerate the cost of those they did purchase.

OMNIBUS RECONCILIATION ACT

Therapy professionals find restraint issues arise in practice. Congress passed the Omnibus Reconciliation Act of 1988 (OBRA) to reform the use of physical restraints in nursing homes in the United States, among other reasons (Omnibus Budget Reconciliation Act of 1987, Pub. L. No. 100-203, 101 Stat. 1330 [OBRA]). OBRA prohibits nursing homes from inappropriately using physical and chemical restraints on nursing home residents for nonmedical purposes. Before OBRA, many nursing homes used restraints for the convenience of nursing home staff. For example, if an individual wandered, the staff did not have to watch that individual if they simply tied the resident to a wheelchair. OBRA sought to stop this kind of abuse.

Under OBRA, nursing homes may not use "as needed" or PRN orders for nursing home residents' restraint use. OBRA only allows the use of restraint as a last resort after the facility completes a comprehensive assessment of the resident and determines less restrictive alternatives failed. According to OBRA, that assessment should include input from the therapists involved in the facility. Even if the facility proves alternatives have failed, numerous other rules apply to protect residents.

DISCRIMINATION LAWS

Discrimination laws raise legal and ethical issues for therapy professionals in their own homes, as well as in relationship to patient issues and fieldwork student issues.

Age

The Age Discrimination in Employment Act of 1967 (Pub. L. 90-202) (ADEA) prohibits employment discrimination against individuals 40 years of age or older. In the therapy context, this prohibition means one must not use age as a factor in employee selection, promotion, and other benefits.

Race

Title VI of the Civil Rights Act of 1964 forbids discrimination against individuals on the basis of race, color, or national origin in participation in benefits of a program that receives or benefits from federal financial assistance (42 USCA § 2000d [West 1995]). Because almost every health care program receives Medicare, Medicaid, or Champus, this nondiscrimination provision applies to health care programs. Therefore, health care practitioners must treat all patients without regard to their race, color, or national origin, and provide the same benefits to all patients.

Title VII of the Civil Rights Act of 1964 prevents employers from discriminating against individuals based on race, color, sex, disabilities, and national origin. This means rehabilitation practitioners must ignore these factors in making hiring, promotion, and other employment-related decisions.

Disability

Title I of the Americans With Disabilities Act (ADA) makes it illegal for employers with 15 or more employees to discriminate against qualified individuals with disabilities in any of the terms, privileges, or conditions of employment. The ADA defines a person with a disability as one who has a physical or mental impairment that substantially limits one or more major life activities, has a record of having such an impairment, or is regarded as having an impairment (29 CFR § 1630[2][g]). A qualified individual with a disability means the individual with a disability meets the requisite skills, experience, and educational requirements of a job and, with or without reasonable accommodations, that individual can perform the essential functions of the job in question (29 CFR § 1630.2[m]; Americans with Disabilities Act § 101[8]).

Under the ADA, employers, at their own expense, must make reasonable accommodations for qualified individuals with disabilities (ADA § 102[b][5]). Reasonable accommodations include procuring needed devices or equipment or changing the way workers perform their work to enable performance despite a disability. However, employers must only provide these reasonable accommodations if they know the applicant or worker is a qualified individual with a disability and if the applicant or worker requests the accommodation (29 CFR §1630.2[o]).

The ADA forbids employers from conducting pre-employment physicals or medical inquiries before extending an offer of employment. It permits employers to conduct preplacement screenings following an offer of employment to determine whether an individual can safely perform the job. An employer may withdraw the offer of employment only if the employer administers a preplacement screening that is job-related and consistent with business necessity. The preplacement screening must also show the individual cannot safely perform the job and the employer could make no accommodation to enable the individual's safe job performance (Appendix to 29 C.F.R. 14, [a], Interpretive Guidelines). These rules intend to prohibit arbitrarily excluding individuals solely because of their disability. Title I of the ADA also prohibits employers from sharing medical information or other information about disabilities with others, including coworkers and prospective employers.

Title III of the ADA makes it illegal to discriminate against individuals with disabilities in access to places of public accommodation and their service that are owned by nongovernment entities or individuals (28 CFR 36 §102). These include doctor's offices, funeral homes, movie theaters, bus stations, amusement parks, museums, restaurants, and just about any other place where the public goes to eat, bank, shop, or engage in commerce or transact business (28 CFR 36 §104). Therapy practitioners need to familiarize themselves with one form of prohibited discrimination that they may encounter. Title III prohibits clinical sites from disclosing a fieldwork student's disability to prospective employers who may call for a reference or others who seek information.

Although physical barriers often prevent access to individuals with disabilities, some of the most significant barriers faced by individuals with disabilities are attitudinal barriers. Whereas Title III provides many building code type regulations, Title III also prevents the type of discrimination caused by attitudinal barriers, which often result from fear, ignorance, stereotypes, and misconceptions about individuals with disabilities.

Fair Housing

In 1989, Congress amended the Fair Housing Act (FHA) ("FHAA") (42 USC § 2601 et seq.), originally intended to prevent housing discrimination against individuals based on race, creed, national origin, and religion, to include individuals with disabilities. Under the FHA, discrimination occurs when a landlord or property owner denies or makes unavailable a property sale or rental because of the disability of the buyer or renter, the intended resident, or any person associated with the person with a disability.

Therapists who involve themselves with making home visits or modifications to the home environment may encounter certain sections of the FHA. Under the FHA, a landlord may not refuse to permit, at the expense of the individual with the disability, reasonable modifications to an existing premises, if the individual with the disability needs the modifications in order to use the dwelling as others do. However, if reasonable, the landlord may condition permission for modification to the apartment on the renter's agreeing to restore the interior to its condition before the modification. The landlord may also condition permission for modifications on provision of a reasonable description of the proposed modification and assurances that workers properly complete the modifications with permits, to code, and in a worker-like fashion.

Under the FHA, the landlord and management company personnel may not refuse to make reasonable accommodations in rules, policies, practices, or services when such accommodations may be necessary to afford an individual with disability equal opportunity to use and enjoy a dwelling unit, including public and common use areas.

FAMILY MEDICAL LEAVE ACT

The Family Medical Leave Act (FMLA) allows employees who have been employed by the employer for at least 12 months and for at least 1,250 hours during the prior 12-month period to take a leave of up to 12 weeks during any 12-month period for certain specified reasons (Table 3-3). Those reasons include birth of a child, placement of a child for

---

Table 3-3

Permissible Reasons for Taking Family Medical Leave

- ◆ The birth of a child and to care for the newborn child
- ◆ The placement of a child with the employee through adoption or foster care and to care for the child
- ◆ To care for the employee's spouse, son, daughter, or parent with a serious health condition
- ◆ Because a serious health condition makes the employee unable to perform one or more of the essential functions of his or her job

---

adoption or foster care, employee need to care for a family member (child, spouse, or parent) with a serious health condition, or because the employee's own serious health condition makes the employee unable to perform the functions of his or her job (29 CFR § 825.100[a]).

A "serious health condition" entitling an employee to family medical leave means an illness, injury, impairment, or physical or mental condition that involves:

1. Inpatient care and the accompanying period of incapacity (i.e., inability to work, attend school, or perform other regular daily activities due to the serious health condition, treatment thereof, or recovery therefrom) or subsequent treatment
2. Three calendar days' absence from normal activities if continuing supervision is required by a health care provider
3. Ongoing care for a chronic or long-term condition that would likely result in a period of incapacity in excess of 3 calendar days if untreated
4. Prenatal care (29 CFR § 825.114)

In addition to the longevity requirement, eligibility to take family medical leave only arises if the employer has 50 or more employees (29 CFR § 825.104). If the employee works at a worksite where the employer employs fewer than 50 employees, the total number of employees employed by that employer within 75 miles of that worksite must be more than 50.

During family medical leave, an employer must maintain the employee's existing level of coverage under a group health plan. At the end of FMLA leave, an employer must take an employee back into the same or an equivalent job with exception only for key employees.

SEXUAL HARASSMENT

Sexual harassment refers to unwanted sexual or gender-based behavior that occurs when one person has formal or informal power over the other (Petrocelli & Repa, 1995). One may exert power based on one's relative position on an organizational chart, one's size, or other reasons.

To fall under the umbrella of sexual harassment, three elements must exist (see Appendix J):

1. The behavior must be unwanted or unwelcome
2. The behavior must be sexual in nature or related to the gender of the person
3. The behavior must occur in the context of a relationship in which one person has more formal power than the other (such as supervisor over an employee) or more informal power (such as one peer over another) (Petrocelli & Repa, 1995)

A variety of conduct may meet this criteria. For example, telling "dirty" jokes, using sexual double entendres in conversation, or giving another worker a hug or kiss may fall within the sexual harassment category.

Sexual harassment exists when one or more conditions occur. The first condition occurs when, explicitly or implicitly, submission to the conduct becomes a term or condition of obtaining employment. For example, one must sleep with the boss to obtain a job.

The second condition occurs where submission or rejection of the conduct becomes a factor in decisions affecting the person's employment. For example, one must sleep with the boss to win a promotion. The conduct has either the purpose or effect of "substantially interfering" with a person's employment.

The conduct must create an "intimidating, hostile, or offensive" work environment. For example, suppose some employees got together and hung nude centerfolds on a department bulletin board. If this behavior intimidated other employees, it might rise to the level of "hostile work environment" (see Appendix J; 29 CFR 1604.11a).

To avoid participating in sexual harassment, before speaking or acting, one can question whether he or she would repeat the same words or actions in front of mom, dad, or a religious or spiritual leader. If no is the answer, do not complete the action or speak the words.

INDIVIDUALS WITH DISABILITIES EDUCATIONAL ACT

The Individuals With Disabilities Educational Act (IDEA) of 1990, Pub L. 101-476, requires public school systems to provide children with disabilities a free, appropriate education in the least restrictive environment. The IDEA mandate requires that schools also provide related services which include, among other services, occupational and physical therapy and speech pathology services. A team creates an individualized educational plan and parents may initiate an appeal through the due process procedures.

THE FAMILY EDUCATIONAL RIGHTS AND PRIVACY ACT

Congress passed the Family Educational Rights and Privacy Act (FERPA), 20 USCA § 1232g & h (1974) (34 CFR § 99), to allow parents and adult students access to their educational records and protect the confidentiality of those records from others. Other than directory information and a few limited exceptions, in order to disclose information from educational records, the parent or adult student must give educational institutions written permission (34 CFR § 99). In the therapy context, this may come to bear on the academic fieldwork program's decision not to inform a fieldwork site of a student's learning disability, for example, should the student not wish to disclose this information.

THE FEDERAL FALSE CLAIMS ACT

The Federal False Claims Act, 31 U.S.C.A. § 3729-3733, allows individuals who discover a fraud against the government and who substantially assist the Department of Justice in prosecuting the case a 15-25% share in the proceeds of the action to recover the damages, civil penalties, and treble damages. The law refers to this as a *Qui Tam* action. This "whistleblower-type" law provides the government with a method of recovering fraudulent claims in health care. Nurses and rehabilitation professionals have successfully used Qui Tam actions in situations where they discovered their employers or others participating in making fraudulent claims.

CONCLUSION

Many legal issues affect those who practice in rehabilitation and many of these issues affect ethical decision making. Therapy practitioners need to familiarize themselves with the rudiments of these legal issues in order to make ethical and legal decisions.

REFERENCES

Areen, J., King, P. A., Goldberg, S., Gostin, L., & Capron, A. M. (1996). *Law, medicine & science*. Westbury, NY: Foundation Press.

Baker, D. B. (1992). *Power quotes*. Detroit, MI: Visible Ink Press.

Biano, E. A., & Hirsh, H. L. (1995). Consent to and refusal of medical treatment. In S. Sanbar (Ed.). *Legal medicine*. St. Louis, MO: Mosby.

Black's Law Dictionary. 5th ed. (1979). St. Paul, MN: West Publishers.

Calloway, S. (1985). *Nursing and the law*. Eau Clare, WI: Professional Education Systems.

Darken, K. J. (1997). Understanding the New Federal Health Care Fraud Legislation. *Florida Bar Journal, 71*, 5 May.

Greaney, T. L. (1997). Night landings on an aircraft carrier: Hospital mergers and antitrust law. *American Journal of Law & Medicine, 23*, 2-3.

Hertfelder, S. D. & Crispen, C. (1990). *Private practice strategies for success*. Rockville, MD: American Occupational Therapy Association.

Hoffman, A. C. (1995). Medical malpractice. In S. Sanbar (Ed.). *Legal medicine*. St. Louis, MO: Mosby.

Hopkins, B. R. & Anderson, B. S. (1990). *The counselor and the law*. Alexandria, VA: American Association for Counseling and Development.

MacDonald M. G., Meyer, K. C., Essig, B. (1985). *Health care law: A practical guide.* New York, NY: Mathew Bender and Associates.

Makar, M. C. (1996). Nursing in Florida: The path to professional liability. *Florida Bar Journal, 70,* 3.

Martin, J. A., & Bjerknes, L. K. (1996). The legal and ethical implications of gag clauses in physician contracts. *American Journal of Law & Medicine, 22,* 4.

Peter, L. J. (1977). *Peter's quotations.* New York, NY: Quill, William Morrow.

Petrocelli, W., & Repa, B. K. (1995). *Sexual harassment on the job.* Berkeley, CA: Nolo Press.

Prosser, W. L. (1971). *Law of torts.* St. Paul, MN: West Publishing Co.

Ranke, B. A., & Moriarty, M. P. (1997). An overview of professional liability in occupational therapy. *American Journal of Occupational Therapy, 51,* 671.

Rosenblatt, R. E., Law, S. A., & Rosenbaum, S. (1997). *Law and the American health care system.* Westbury, NY: Foundation Press.

Salcido, R. (1996). Applications of the False Claims Act-Knowledge: Standard: What one must know to be held liable under the act. *The Health Lawyer, 8,* 1.

Stromberg, C., Hagarty, D. J., Leibenluft, R. F., et. al. (1988). *The psychologist's legal handbook.* Washington, DC: Council for National Register of Health Service Providers in Psychology.

Weinstein, M. M. (1991). *The law of federal income taxation.* Deerfield, IL: Callaghan and Company.

CASES

- *Arizona v. Maricopa County Medical Society,* 457 U.S. 332 (1982)
- *Board of Regents v. Taborsky,* 648 So. 2d 748 (Fla. 2d DCA 1994)
- *Northern Pacific Railway v. United States,* 365 U.S. 1, 4-5 (1958)

STATUTES, REGULATIONS, AND OTHER LEGAL CITES

- Restatement of Law, Agency (2nd ed.) § 220 (2) 1957

- Rev. Rul. 87-41, CB 1987-1, 296
- Appendix to 29 C.F.R. 14, (a), Interpretive Guidelines
- 29 CFR § 1630(2)(g)
- 29 CFR § 1630.2(m); Americans with Disabilities Act § 101(8)
- ADA § 102(b)(5)
- 29 CFR §1630.2(o)
- Appendix to 29 C.F.R. 14, (a), Interpretive Guidelines
- 28 CFR 36 §102
- 28 CFR 36 §104
- 29 CFR 1604.11a
- Fair Housing Act, 42 USC § 2601 et seq.
- Individuals With Disabilities Educational Act of 1990, Pub L. 101-476
- Fla Stat § 812.081
- Fla Stat § 688.002(4)
- Fla Stat § 688.003(1)
- HCFA Health Insurance Manual for Home Health Care § 106.1 7/92
- Department of Health and Human Services, Regulations on Protection of Human Services, 45 CFR 46 (1994)
- Health Care Portability and Accountability Act of 1996, Public Law 104-191 (1996)
- Omnibus Budget Reconciliation Act of 1987, Pub. L. No. 100-203, 101 Stat. 1330 (OBRA)
- Title VI of the Civil Act Rights of 1964, 42 USCA § 2000d (West 1995)
- The Age Discrimination in Employment Act of 1967, (Pub. L. 90-202)
- Family Educational Rights and Privacy Act, 20 USCA § 1232g & h, (1974) (FERPA) 34 CFR § 99

4

Ethics and Managed Care

When morality comes up against profit, it is seldom profit that loses.
Congresswoman Shirley Chisholm, quoted in Baker, 1992

Why write about managed care in a book about ethics in rehabilitation? Managed care engenders many ethical issues for health care providers working in rehabilitation. The very notions that support managed care threaten patient autonomy, informed consent, a plethora of patient rights, veracity (through acts of omission), justice, and paternalism.

Until the proliferation of technology in health care occurred, hospital lengths of stay varied little. In many parts of the United States in the 1940s, women giving birth stayed in the hospital the same length of time as individuals recovering from heart attacks (Gordon, 1992). Sophisticated tests and procedures could not increase the length of stay because they did not yet exist.

With the explosion of technology in health care, individuals seeking hospital care found themselves facing a plethora of procedures, from computer-assisted tomography (CAT scan) to magnetic resonance imaging (MRI) and a host of others. With these advances in technology came increased costs and longer hospital stays. Suddenly, doctors could keep people alive who previously found themselves with no chance of survival. However, this recurring miracle cost a great deal of money (Sultz & Young, 1997).

For a long time, insurance companies followed their custom and paid the costs of these procedures almost without question. Essentially, insurance companies reimbursed health care providers for whatever charges they billed, with some minor exceptions. This practice occurred until the climate began to change for government-run programs, such as Medicare and Medicaid, as well as private insurance programs.

THE CHANGING FACE OF MEDICARE

As expenses crested, government tried to slow the growth of health care costs by implementing the diagnostic-related groups (DRG) system. Under the DRG system, Medicare no longer paid hospitals based on the full amount billed. Instead, Medicare reimbursed hospitals a prospective set amount determined by the patient's diagnosis on admission (Baldor, 1996).

For example, suppose Mrs. O'Leary ruptures her left widget joint and requires a surgical repair. Under the DRG system, the facility would know on admission the exact amount of money and number of days for which Medicare will reimburse. Assume for illustration purposes Medicare reimburses 5 days for a ruptured widget. If the facility could discharge Mrs. O'Leary in 3 days, thereby spending less than the prescribed amount, it made money. If Mrs. O'Leary stayed in the hospital longer than the 5 days allowed, the facility lost money.

As a result of the DRG system, hospitals discharged patients much more rapidly and much earlier in their convalescence. At the same time, advances in technology and medical research increased the chances of sicker patients surviving more complex medical situations. Technological advances allowed patients to leave the hospital taking life-saving devices with them. Many of these patients still required rehabilitation and many other services.

Initially, therapists saw the DRG system as the doom of their professions. However, reality painted a different picture. The economic pressure from the DRG system forced hospitals to discharge patients faster, but the patients were still in need of rehabilitation and other care. In response to the increased numbers of patients in need of rehabilitation and other medical services outside acute care hospitals, three events occurred.

First, many facilities opened DRG-exempt rehabilitation units to serve their patients and others outside the acute care setting. Existing rehabilitation hospitals increased their patient capacities, and new free-standing rehabilitation hospitals opened their doors for business for the first time.

Second, long-term care experienced an unprecedented boom, especially in rehabilitation. Construction of long-term care facilities increased sharply. Existing long-term care facilities expanded their rehabilitation programs to compete with the new facilities' rehabilitation programs. With job opportunities seemingly endless and boundless, many occupational therapists, physical therapists, speech pathologists, respiratory therapists, and other health professionals found a home in the long-term care boom market.

Third, home health care experienced a dramatic surge in the number of patients and, consequently, demand for rehabilitation services. Hospitals developed their own home care units and other new home care companies ventured into business.

Creative therapists and administrators developed other DRG-exempt programs, including psychiatric and alcohol and drug rehabilitation units. These programs gave therapists even more job opportunities.

Thus, the DRG system did not actually cut costs. Over time, the DRG system merely shifted costs from acute hospital to long-term and home health care (Rosenblatt, Law, & Rosenbaum, 1997).

MANAGED CARE

At the same time, health care costs increased in the Medicare program and health care costs increased for everyone (Rosenblatt, Law, & Rosenbaum, 1997; Sultz & Young, 1997). Beginning in the late 1970s and early 1980s, employers watched as their employee health insurance premiums began an upward spiral. Many employers responded to these cost increases by cutting benefits provided by the plans, raising deductibles and copayments required by the plans, or raising the percentage amount of the premium paid by the employee (AOTA Managed Care Team, 1996). Some employers stopped paying for health insurance benefits for employees, offering an option to pay the cost of their health insurance through the company's group plan. During this time, premiums for individual health insurance policies soared as well.

Employers and business and trade groups sought financially reasonable alternatives and solutions. Health maintenance organizations (HMOs) and preferred provider organizations (PPOs) emerged as alternatives to higher-priced medical insurance plans. Tracing their origins back to the 1930s, when Kaiser Construction Company developed the HMO concept for its workers' building government projects, in the early 1970s only a handful of HMOs existed (Rosenblatt, Law, & Rosenbaum, 1997; Stromberg et al., 1988). In 1973, Congress passed the Health Maintenance Act, which fostered the development of HMOs and required most employers offering health plans to offer federally qualified HMOs as an option (Stromberg et al., 1988; Sultz & Young, 1997). This created a minimum standard for HMOs to follow in order to meet the "federally qualified" designation (Sultz & Young, 1997). Once confined to a handful of cities and programs, as the 1980s moved along, many people joined HMOs and new ones opened in different parts of the country.

Many people still could not afford health insurance. Others complained about access to health care or quality of care, while employers complained about the high cost of health insurance premiums. Thus began the crisis in private health care.

President Clinton ran for office in the 1992 presidential election on a platform that promised a national health care plan to solve the health care crisis. President Clinton charged the first lady, Hillary Rodham Clinton, with the task of developing the national health care plan. Despite much effort, the government could not come up with a plan that would please everyone and that Congress would pass (Rosenblatt, Law, & Rosenbaum, 1997). America mourned the death of the government's national health insurance plan.

With the death of the government's plan, the problem continued. Private insurance companies took over, developing and modifying their own plans, which soon gained popularity as "managed care plans."

Managed care refers to a system of cost-containment principles in which the payer of services (or insurer) controls both the recipient's use of health care and the cost of that care (AOTA Managed Care Team, 1996; Baldor, 1996; Burton & Popok, 1998; Rosenblatt, Law, & Rosenbaum, 1997; Sultz & Young, 1997). The control or oversight may occur prospectively by gatekeepers, case managers, and specified service providers, or retrospectively through utilization review, termination of provider contracts, and second opinion (Baldor, 1996; Burton & Popok, 1998; DeMarco & Wolfe, 1995; Sultz & Young, 1997; Weiner & de Lissovoy, 1993).

Their fourfold goal:

1. To continue to provide some level of health care services
2. To stop the cost of health care from rising exponentially
3. To keep health care premiums affordable for employers
4. To make money

OTHER TRENDS TOWARD MANAGED CARE

As the payers began to take matters into their own hands, employers responded. Many employers were accustomed to offering their employees a choice of several different health insurance plans. As the costs of traditional indemnity plans—those that paid a fee for health care services provided to patients—skyrocketed, employers began to encourage employees to shift to the cheaper HMOs and PPOs it offered, both falling under the managed care umbrella. Employers increased the employee portion of the insurance premiums for indemnity plans, raised deductibles to an unaffordable amount for most workers, and some even stopped offering the high-priced indemnity plans (AOTA Managed Care Team, 1996; Rosenblatt, Law, & Rosenbaum, 1997).

As the health care crisis developed, a crisis in workers' compensation also grew. Because a large part of workers' compensation's costs comes from payment for health care costs, as private health insurance costs reached for the sky, so did workers' compensation premiums. Many workers' compensation systems responded to this crisis by putting in place fee schedules, which dictate the amount of reimbursement for specific covered services (DeMarco & Wolfe, 1995). Currently, workers' compensation's new trend places injured workers in HMOs or other managed care arrangements for their medical care. "Twenty-four hour coverage," another trend on the horizon, covers workers' health (as the name implies—24 hours a day), covering injuries or illnesses both off the job and on the job.

Since the early 1980s when it began in Miami, FL, as an experiment to cut Medicare costs, industry watchers have seen an increase in Medicare recipient membership in HMOs (Rosenblatt, Law, & Rosenbaum, 1997). In some parts of the country where this option is available, Medicare recipients can elect membership in Medicare HMOs. Medicare HMOs often use aggressive marketing campaigns to sell memberships especially geared to healthy, younger Medicare recipients (Rosenblatt, Law, & Rosenbaum, 1997). Membership in Medicare HMOs looks enticing to those on a fixed income, especially as the Medicare HMOs often provide additional benefits not covered by traditional Medicare, such as eyeglasses and medications. The government's Medicare program pays the HMOs a set amount for taking charge of the individual member's managed care arrangement.

Another trend involves Medicaid and HMOs. The Medicaid program provides medical care for the medically indigent. The federal government sets the minimum benefits and the states, which administer the Medicaid program, may add to the basic benefits, should they choose to participate in Medicaid. Over the last several years, the federal government allowed the states to try new means of delivering health care. States obtained "waivers" from the federal government giving them the right to start alternative Medicaid programs branching out into the managed care arena (Stromberg, Loeb, Thomen, & Krause, 1996). Some states choose to place Medicaid recipients in HMOs as a way of lowering costs (Baldor, 1996).

As workers' compensation, Medicare, Medicaid, and employers began to utilize managed care, HMOs gained in strength, numbers, and members. With all these systems and programs relying on managed care, how can managed care payers control health care costs? The tools of managed care include the following:

- Gatekeeping
- Capitation
- Case management
- Gag rules

Gatekeeping

Managed care often uses gatekeepers to help control health care costs. Gatekeepers monitor the patient's access to health care services. In theory, gatekeepers decide what care the patient needs and keeps the gate open wide enough for the patient to obtain only those services (Weiner & de Lissovoy, 1993). Instead of ordering a menu of tests and other interventions for the patient, the gatekeeper orders only what he or she believes necessary for the patient to receive. The gatekeeper provides what he or she sees as adequate care—not necessarily optimal care. Often the primary care physician fills the role of gatekeeper (Burton & Popok, 1998).

The gatekeeper controls the patient's access to health care. A visit to the gatekeeper physician, the first step in the process, begins the treatment game. Patients who require care from other health care providers must first see their gatekeeper physician. The gatekeeper controls referrals to other physicians and specialists as well as therapy providers. The gatekeeper physician determines what care the patient needs and authorizes only that care without regard for the patient's autonomy (Beauchamp & Childress, 1994; Gunderson, 1997).

Capitation

"It is difficult to get a man to understand something when his salary depends on his not understanding it."
Upton Sinclair, quoted in Gardner & Reese, 1996

One cannot discuss gatekeepers without discussing capitation. Some insurers control costs by paying the primary care physician, or gatekeeper, a lump sum payment, per patient, per month, to cover all services the patients receive (Burton & Popok, 1998; Weiner & de Lissovoy, 1993). The industry calls this lump sum payment method *capitation*.

The gatekeeper physician pays for the patient services he or she orders out of that lump sum, or capitated amount. In theory, the patient pool includes a mix of sick individuals who use more health care services and healthy individuals who rarely require health care services (Rosenblatt, Law, & Rosenbaum, 1997). Should the gatekeeper physician spend less money than the allotted lump sum, he or she makes money. Should he or she spend more money than the allotted lump sum, he or she loses money.

Depending on the nature of the plan, payment for therapy services often comes out of the capitated amount the gatekeeper physician receives. Because physicians make more money for authorizing less treatment, the bottom line may affect some gatekeepers' judgment as to which services that patient really needs. This presents an ethical dilemma to physicians. Do they provide more care to the patient and make less money or less care to the patient, as the HMO wants them to do, and make more money (Gunderson, 1997)? Some payers provide gatekeeper physicians with bonuses at the end of the year as additional incentives to keep the number of referrals to specialists low, adding to the gatekeeper's ethical dilemma. Others refuse to renew the contracts of gatekeepers who make too many referrals (Burton & Popok, 1998). This gatekeeper's ethical dilemma may affect both the number and type of referrals therapy professionals receive.

Another type of capitation occurs in long-term

care. When Medicare HMO members enter long-term care facilities, the managed care companies pay the facilities a capitated or lump sum rate for services rather than an individual amount for each service provided.

Case Management

Managed care payers employ case managers as another way of controlling costs. Usually nurses, and sometimes social workers or therapists, case managers ("CCM" following a case manager's name indicates certification as a certified case manager) help control costs by reviewing treatment plans, determining patient needs, and negotiating with providers for cost-effective services, supplies, and equipment (DeMarco & Wolfe, 1995). Case managers also coordinate care so the right hand knows what the left hand is doing. Some case managers work inhouse, over the phone, or for payers, while others work out in the field, with face-to-face patient contact. Case managers concern themselves with the bottom line while trying to provide the patient with the care he or she needs at the best possible price.

Gag Rules

Gag rules prevent a health care provider from discussing treatment alternatives with patients. Formal gag rules come from clauses in the contract between the health care provider and the HMO or other managed care organization (AOTA Managed Care Team, 1996). Informal gag rules occur where, for example, therapists are encouraged "to keep their mouths shut" about a particular practice they encounter in order not to risk losing the patient, client, or referral source. Although not a contractual issue, with informal gag rules, other threats hang in the background, such as losing one's job.

In theory, gag rules keep costs down by limiting the choices a patient can make regarding his or her health care (Rosenblatt, Law, & Rosenbaum, 1997). For example, suppose a patient arrives at his gatekeeper physician's office with chest pains. The physician examines the patient and decides the patient needs to remove himself from stress for a few days. In the old days, before managed care, the physician might have ordered an echocardiogram, a cardiac stress test, and a full set of blood work. In

this case, the gag rule prohibits the physician gatekeeper from discussing these other more costly alternatives with the patient. In some contracts, gag rules forbid therapists or other health care providers from discussing their fees with patients and other therapists.

Some states have passed, or tried to pass, laws to make gag clauses illegal. However, under the Employee Retirement Income Security Act (ERISA), a federal law, these state laws do not apply to self-insured managed care plans (Stromberg et al., 1988). Self-insured managed care plans include plans that, instead of purchasing insurance, insure their own risk and hire an administrator to administer the plan only. Until Congress acts, the gag rules remain in effect if included in contracts between health care providers and self-insured funds (Burton & Popok, 1998).

IMPACT OF MANAGED CARE ON PRACTICE

At the dawn of the institution of DRGs, therapists feared the worst. Many thought jobs would go by the wayside. Reality brought a booming market with more jobs than graduates could handle. Managed care once again changed the way therapists do business (Table 4-1).

Decreased Days, Dollars, Number of Treatments

Managed care brings both positive and negative changes to therapy practice. Many therapists can readily recite the major drawback of managed care—decreased days, dollars, and treatments. Under managed care, patient care no longer lasts forever. The payer limits the number of days of inpatient and outpatient care, as well as the number of days of therapy.

The dollars part of the equation means therapists see reimbursement amounts decreasing along with the number of treatments allowed, either because of the limits of the individual's managed care plan or lack of authorization from the gatekeeper. The payer may only cover a limited number of visits according to the managed care plan. Even if the plan covers more visits, the therapist may find only a limited

---

Table 4-1

Impact of Managed Care on Practice

- ◆ Decreased days, dollars, number of treatments
- ◆ Focus on outcomes and function
- ◆ Introduction of practice parameters/critical pathways
- ◆ Capitation
- ◆ Case managers, physicians, and other gatekeepers
- ◆ Change in the face of private practice
- ◆ Gag rules
- ◆ Change to program management
- ◆ Questionable ethical practice

---

number of authorized treatment sessions with which to work.

Focus on Outcomes and Function

The focus on outcomes brings a positive change to therapy practice. Therapists now find themselves responsible for their patient's outcomes. This added accountability gives the therapist more of a stake in the outcome of the patient and fosters a partnership between the therapist and the patient. The emphasis on outcomes encourages data gathering and simplifies one aspect of clinic work. Clinically based outcomes research strengthens the profession, adds to the body of knowledge of one's profession, and justifies what health and rehabilitation professionals do.

The focus on outcomes also promotes a focus on function as an outcome. Therapists now look to functional outcomes rather than performance components or pieces of a goal. They can measure the patient's progress by looking at how the patient now functions in his or her day-to-day life. The focus shifts to making a difference in the individual's life.

Practice Parameters/Critical Pathways

Practice parameters and critical pathways serve as another reminder that things have changed as a result of managed care. Some view this as a good change because of the streamlined documentation and set standards everyone must follow. Others criticize this way of practicing as "cookbook" treatment that removes the element of creativity and ingenuity from the therapist and individuality from the patient.

Legally, the limited documentation under the critical pathway system may not provide adequate protection for therapists in the event of a threatening malpractice action. Documentation should always include the tasks done with a patient in case one needs to justify one's actions at a later date under very different circumstances.

Capitation

As previously discussed, physicians face an ethical dilemma with capitation because the less care they provide, the more money they make. As a result of this dilemma, therapists may not have enough authorized visits to treat the patient properly. This may lead to issues of patient abandonment should the therapist discharge a patient prematurely due to lack of authorized visits combined with the patient's inability to assume the costs or contractual prohibitions against patients doing so.

In long-term care, Medicare managed care providers may provide a capitated rate for therapy separate from the daily bed rate. In one case, a facility received $50 per day for therapy with instructions to spend it on therapy "any way they saw fit." This capitation arrangement placed pressure on the therapists to see more patients at one time, in some cases compromising the quality of care. This also added pressure to use "cheaper" providers, including students, unlicensed aides, and rehab techs—in some cases an illegal move according to state licensure laws. Ironically, the pressure of this capitation arrangement also limits the time allowable for supervising these unlicensed personnel.

Capitation may also encourage, consciously or unconsciously, discrimination in care, with patients under capitation receiving less care and poorer quality care than those whose insurance carriers pay a higher reimbursement amount. Finally, capitation pressures therapists to limit the amount spent on treatment and may therefore eliminate the use of certain equipment with these patients.

Case Managers, Physicians, and Other Gatekeepers

Case managers, physicians, and other gatekeepers, as nontherapists, dictate to therapists what they can and cannot do and for how long they can do it. Often these gatekeepers dictate their wishes from another location, without ever examining the patient. This can lower the quality of care and tempt health and rehabilitation professionals to place their standards of practice in the hands of the nontherapist. Therapists can also face issues of patient abandonment should the gatekeeper seek to discontinue therapy before standards of practice or patient need dictate.

Gatekeepers pressure therapists for results. They authorize "adequate" care—not optimum care. Case managers look for the best care for the least cost. The case manager "game" sounds similar to the television show *Name That Tune*—"I can rehab that patient in 8 days..." "I can rehab that patient in 7 days..." "Rehab that patient!"

In some situations therapists find pressure from their employers to exaggerate the patient's condition to show better outcomes. If the case manager likes the results, he or she will send more patients in that direction.

Some may find themselves pressured to discharge patients too early, risking patient safety and losing the ability to continue seeing the patient due to cost constraints. Discrimination in care may also occur. If other patients bring in higher reimbursement amounts, these patients may move to the top of the priority list for care, leaving the patients with care plans providing lower reimbursement at the bottom. At the same time, the pressure for results and outcomes looms overhead.

The Changing Face of Private Practice

Private practitioners find the transition to managed care difficult. Many therapy practitioners find selling their practices an easier choice than coping with declining dollars in health care. Others form alliances with fellow therapy practitioners to position themselves to bid for large managed care contracts. Those who did not jump on the managed care bandwagon early found themselves closed out of provider panels.

Hospitals and large health care corporations continue to buy out successful therapy practices in the mergers and acquisitions game. Some private practitioners just do not want to practice under managed care because the focus seems to have shifted away from patient care.

Gag Rules

Like physicians, therapists covered by gag rule provisions may not discuss treatment alternatives with patients. Without the ability to discuss alternatives, the gag rule interferes with the therapist's ability to obtain informed consent and respect the patient's autonomy. If therapists cannot discuss appropriate treatment alternatives with patients, this can interfere with the therapist's ability to provide appropriate care, educate the patient, and appropriately plan for the patient's discharge.

The gag rule's prohibitions may influence therapist judgment by steering the therapist to another treatment under the guise of proper care. Patients receiving care under a gag rule may also face discrimination in care, as other patients not covered by a gag clause receive an appropriate treatment and they do not.

Change to Program Management

Until recent years, most health care facilities used a form of management on a department level now referred to as departmentalization. Under departmentalization in rehabilitation, three departments existed side by side: an occupational therapy (OT) department, a physical therapy (PT) department, and a speech and language pathology (SLP) department. With the pressure on facilities to streamline and cut costs, many facilities switched from departmentalization to program management. Program management divides the organizations by programs. Instead of a chief or director of OT, PT, and SLP, the facility now has a program manager for each program. For example, a facility might have a spinal cord program manager, a work rehabilitation program manager, and a neurology program manager.

With this system in place, program managers find themselves supervising individuals from different professional backgrounds and may lack an understanding of that professional's role in treatment. The program manager may find it difficult to evaluate a subordinate's performance if he or she lacks a clear picture of that professional's role.

The program management form of organization may also make the transition from student to therapist difficult owing to the absence of role models in the same field. It may also interfere with opportunities for mentorship within one's own profession and interfere with on-the-job learning experiences from peers.

Questionable Ethical Practice

The changes brought on by managed care contribute a plethora of questionable ethical practices to an already existing field. In health care, whenever one finds reimbursement at risk, ethics and morals are at risk. Section II of this book contains numerous illustrations of actual questionable ethical practices.

CURRENT AND FUTURE DEVELOPMENTS IN MEDICARE MANAGED CARE

Although Medicare began its trek into the managed care arena with the introduction of optional Medicare HMO membership, it has not stopped there. Recently, three other changes went into place to continue to cut costs and control care. These include salary equivalency, the prospective payment system in long-term care, and the $1,500 cap on all outpatient services provided outside the hospital setting and all home health care services.

Salary equivalency for physical therapists went into place before speech pathology and occupational therapy. By the time the government developed and announced regulations for occupational therapy and speech pathology salary equivalency, the prospective payment system made salary equivalency a moot proposition. The prospective payment system removed salary equivalency's bang. It no longer mat-

tered once the payment focus shifted from hourly monetary limits paid for the therapist's services to a prospective payment per individual patient.

On the other hand, the prospective payment system and Medicare's $1,500 cap created more of an uproar. Seeking other ways to cut Medicare costs, Congress passed legislation to cap outpatient occupational therapy services at $1,500, and physical therapy and speech pathology combined to $1,500. (At the time of this writing, a bill was introduced in Congress to repeal the caps. Because health care regulations change so rapidly, readers should check with their professional organizations for the most up-to-date regulations and read the newspaper.) The cap, according to the Balanced Budget Act of 1997, applies to all outpatient therapy services, except those provided through a hospital.

Prospective Payment System

"I cannot and will not cut my conscience to fit this year's fashions."
Lillian Hellman to the Committee on Un-American Activities, House of Representatives, May 19, 1952, quoted in Baker, 1992

The most profound recent change in Medicare put the prospective payment system in place. Congress passed the prospective payment system as part of the Balanced Budget Act of 1997 to save Medicare dollars. Over a 4-year period, the prospective payment system shifts reimbursement in long-term care from cost-based reporting to a prospective payment system. No longer will long-term care facilities receive additional reimbursement for their operating costs and no longer will rehabilitation services receive additional separate reimbursement. The new prospective payment system assigns payment amounts prospectively based on the amount of services the patient needs. The Balanced Budget Act's changes may tempt therapists with ethical dilemmas because of the new methods used to set the amount of therapy a patient receives.

All of the "players" in the facility evaluate the patient using their individual evaluations. The results are incorporated into the Minimum Data Set (MDS) II, including the total number of minutes OT, PT, and SLP plan to treat the patient. From the MDS, providers derive an activities of daily living (ADL) score, which specifies how much nursing care the patient requires.

The facility takes the MDS data, including the total number of minutes of therapy, from the MDS and translates it into a resource utilization grouping (RUGS) formula (RUGS III). The RUGS III assigns a RUGS group level to the patient. The RUGS group levels range from the lowest level, called PA1 (basically an independent patient in need of no therapy and no nursing care), to RUC (rehabilitation ultra high-level "C"), the highest of the 44 levels. The severity of the condition or the amount of therapy or nursing required forms the basis for the range of the 44 levels. The assigned level determines the amount of money, in the form of a per diem rate, that Medicare will reimburse the facility for that particular patient's care. This rate may change based on the patient's subsequent MDS evaluations (Colmar, 1998).

Like all documentation, the MDS is a legal document. Those who fill out the form must sign the sections of the MDS they fill out. If therapists exaggerate their characterization of the patient's condition or the number of minutes they treat the patient, they can find themselves facing charges of Medicare fraud. The prospective payment system now permits payment for group therapy under certain specified circumstances and also allows for maintenance therapy on a limited basis in certain specific circumstances. Unfortunately, many providers of rehabilitation services initially responded to changes from the Balanced Budget Act amendments by cutting salaries and laying off clinicians. History may indicate to clinicians, administrators, educators, and students that the Balanced Budget Act amendments may not signal doom and despair for therapists, but may open up new opportunities for the future.

CONCLUSION

As readers examine the steps taken by Medicare and other insurer/payers to control costs, they will see how these steps continue to present ethical dilemmas in their professional practice. Because these regulations change often, therapists must stay current with the changes. The internet provides a great resource for this purpose (see Appendix Q).

REFERENCES

American Occupational Therapy Association Managed Care Team. (1996). *Managed care: an occupational therapy sourcebook.* Bethesda, MD: AOTA.

Baker, D. B. (1992). *Power quotes.* Detroit, MI: Visible Ink Press.

Baldor, R. A. (1996). *Managed care made simple.* Cambridge, MA: Blackwell Science.

Beauchamp, T. L., & Childress. (1994). *Principles of biomedical ethics.* New York: Oxford University Press.

Burton, D. N. & Popok, M. S. (1998). Managed care 101. *Florida Bar Journal, 72,* 4:26.

Cohen, A. (1995). Practice organizations and joint ventures. In S. Sanbar (Ed.). *Legal medicine.* St. Louis, MO: Mosby.

Colmar, M. (1998). Private consultations and conversations regarding the prospective payment system.

DeMarco, W. J., & Wolfe, K. (1995). Managed care concepts in the delivery of disability management services to industry. In D. E. Shrey & M. Lecerte (Eds.). *Principle and practices of disability management in industry.* Winter Park, FL: GR Press.

Gardner, J. W., & Reese, F. G. (1996). *Wit & wisdom.* New York: W. W. Norton & Company.

Gordon, J. (1992). How America's health care fell ill. *American Heritage,* May/June, 49-66.

Gunderson, M. (1997). Eliminating conflicts of managed care organizations through disclosure and consent. *Journal of Law, Medicine & Ethics, 25,* 92-98.

Rosenblatt, R. E., Law, S. A., & Rosenbaum, S. (1997). *Law and the American health care system.* Westbury, NY: Foundation Press.

Stromberg, C., Loeb, L., Thomen, S., & Krause, J. (1996). State initiatives in health care reform. In J. Hall (Ed.). The psychologist's legal update. *National Register of Health Service Providers in Psychology,* January.

Stromberg C., et. al. (1988). *The psychologist's legal handbook.* Washington, DC: Council for National Register of Health Service Providers in Psychology.

Sultz, H. A., & Young, K. M. (1997). *Health care USA: understanding its organization and delivery.* Gaithersburg, MD: Aspen.

Weiner, J., & de Lissovoy, G. (1993). Razing the tower of babel: A taxonomy for managed care and health insurance plans. *Journal of Health Politics, Policy and Law, 75.*

5

Ethics and the Law: The Interface

Ethical right is largely abstract; legal right is mostly concrete. Ethical right the just man wishes to be established; legal right is already established ... One is founded on power, on might; the other on justice, on equality. One appeals to the sword to settle matters, the other appeals to the judgment of men.

Charles E. Sprading, quoted in Seldes, 1972

As previously mentioned, today's health care environment presents many ethical and legal challenges for health care providers. Sometimes the course one chooses appears as a straightforward decision. Other times a course of action may raise ethical issues. Still other situations raise an "Is this legal?" flag for the health care practitioner. Sometimes the ethical action one chooses conflicts with the law. Conversely, a decision based on the letter of the law may not abide by one's ethical and moral beliefs.

Four paradigms outline the relationship between an ethical action and a legal action. When faced with an ethical dilemma, one may choose a course of action that is both legal and ethical; legal but not ethical; not legal or ethical; or ethical but not legal. The penalty one may face varies with the action and approach one chooses (Figure 5-1).

Penalties for illegal actions or behaviors differ from penalties for unethical behaviors or actions, although some overlap exists. Professional associations enforce their codes of ethics, each through their own process. Penalties resulting from the enforcement procedures for ethical violations can include loss of membership in one's professional association; loss of certification or other privilege; public or private reprimand; public censure; report to the licensure board, which can assess a fine for the same

unethical behavior; report to the certification board; or termination. Professional associations often publish public reprimand and censure in one of their professional publications to notify the other members.

Conversely, legal matters carry some different penalties. Depending on the legal offense, one might face fines or other monetary damages, including punitive damages (assessed as a punishment), compensatory damages (assessed to compensate for a harm), or restitution (designed to restore the harmed party to their previous position). If a therapist breaks the law by committing Medicare fraud, for example, the therapist may face imprisonment. Injunction, another penalty, occurs when in response to a request from a party to a legal matter, a judge orders an individual to stop committing some particular act so the parties may return to their previous position. For example, a court might issue an injunction to prevent a long-term care facility from discharging patients solely because they have Alzheimer's disease, which is in violation of the Americans With Disabilities Act (ADA).

As with ethical problems, legal problems can also lead to revocation or suspension of one's license by the licensure board's action. As discussed in the previous chapter, most licensure laws specify certain forbidden behaviors, which often include the commission of a felony crime or a crime of dishonesty.

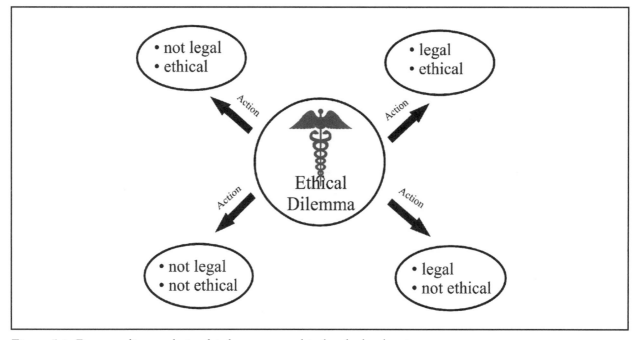

Figure 5-1. Four paradigms: relationship between an ethical and a legal action.

Based on one's behavior, the licensure board may suspend or revoke one's license, or place one's license in a probationary status while assessing specific terms one must meet in order to regain his or her full license. For example, the licensure board might require the therapist to work under the supervision of another therapist for a period of time, or to have progress notes and other documentation cosigned for a period of time. Finally, breaking the law can lead to termination, especially if an individual loses his or her license. Because licensure boards function to protect the public, they often provide a mechanism for notifying the public of its actions when they find an individual violated its rules under the law.

See Table 5-1 for a comparison of legal and ethical penalties.

CASE STUDY

The following case study illustrates the four paradigms and the penalties that may result from the chosen behavior:

Mary recently graduated from school and has a temporary license. In the long-term care facility where she works, she walks into a patient's room to begin to treat the patient and finds the patient on the *floor. Mary has a history of facing reprimands from her supervisor for failing to lock the wheelchair.*

Legal and Ethical Response

Mary responds in a manner that is both legal and ethical when she immediately rings the call bell for help. She follows this up, if necessary, by attempting to alert others in the hall outside the door to the room. She reassures the patient if the patient is alert. Mary recognizes both a legal and ethical duty to get help and reassure the patient. In acting this way, she puts the patient's needs first. She abides by the ethical principle of beneficence by pursuing a duty to help the patient. Her actions support the legal duty owed to the patient by a reasonable, prudent, similarly trained health care professional.

Possible Penalties

None. Mary acted ethically and legally.

Legal but Unethical Response

Mary responds in a legal but not ethical manner. She checks to make sure the patient has not broken any bones. She asks the patient if she is in any pain, to which the patient replies "No." Seeing no injury,

---

Table 5-1

Legal and Ethical Penalties

FEATURE	LAW	ETHICS
Comprised of:	Federal statutes	Standards of practice
	State statutes	Codes of ethics
	State regulations	Social values
	Federal regulations	Religious values
	Case law	Cultural values
	(Licensure laws)	Moral values
Penalties:	Fines	Fines
	Monetary damages (punitive, compensatory, or restitution)	Loss of professional privilege, license, or certification
	Imprisonment	Relinquishment of membership in professional organization
	Injunctions	Reprimand—public or private
	Revocation or suspension of license	Censure—usually public
	Publication of revocation or suspension of license	Publication of the ethical violation and penalty imposed
	License placed in probationary status	Report to licensure or certification board
	Termination	Termination

Mary assists the patient back into her chair. Mary keeps the incident to herself because she fears she will get in trouble. Although some may disagree, Mary has acted legally. She committed no crime by her actions and brought no harm to the patient. However, by her actions, Mary showed that she places her needs above the patient's needs. She disregarded the facility policy that requires one to report incidents such as this one and covers up the incident, violating the principle of veracity by omission.

Possible Penalties

If her supervisor discovers her actions, Mary will face reprimand from her supervisor and could lose her job. The patient, supervisor, coworkers, or facility representatives could report Mary's behavior to the professional association's ethics enforcement body for violation of the professional code of ethics. If reported, Mary will have to defend her actions to the ethics enforcement body. As a result of the ethics enforcement body's action, Mary could face a public or private reprimand, find her membership revoked, and lose her reputation. Further, if the ethics body finds a violation and reports it to the licensing board, Mary may have to defend herself before the licensing board and face possible revocation, suspension, or supervision of her license on a probationary sta-

tus. The licensing board may also notify the public of its actions.

Ethical but Illegal Response

Mary's ethical but illegal response begins with her failing to ask the patient whether she hurt herself as a result of the fall. Without regard for the patient's safety, Mary, realizing she needs to help the patient, improperly lifts the patient, dislocating her arm in the process. She then reports the incident to her supervisor. In this response scenario, Mary realizes a duty to help the patient, according to the principle of beneficence. She realizes she has a duty to report the incident to her supervisor and she abides by the principle of veracity by truthfully reporting. However, her conduct raises the legal flag because by her actions she fell below the standard of care of a reasonable, prudent health care professional. A reasonable, prudent health care practitioner would know how to lift the patient properly or realize the need for help to lift the patient. By physically hurting the patient, the therapist's actions are negligent and supportive of the patient's position should the patient file a lawsuit for malpractice. State licensure boards also may conclude that this conduct falls below the standard of care contained in the state's practice act.

Possible Penalties

Because Mary's actions fell below the standard of care of a reasonable, prudent therapist and harmed the patient, Mary will likely face a malpractice lawsuit, which she has a good chance of losing. As a result of the malpractice action against her, Mary's malpractice rates will increase. Her supervisor may find herself implicated for failing to supervise Mary properly. Mary may not receive her permanent license as a result of her actions or the licensure board may require her to practice under supervision on a probationary license.

Unethical and Illegal Response

In the unethical and illegal scenario, Mary simply picks up the patient, dislocating the patient's arm in the process, and leaves the room without telling anyone. By failing to consider the patient's need, Mary harmed the patient, thereby violating the ethical principle of nonmaleficence. Mary violated the principle of veracity by failing to report the incident and her involvement in it. Mary's actions fell below the standard of care of a reasonable, prudent health care professional and she will probably find herself liable for malpractice.

Possible Penalties

In light of Mary's imprudent care, the harm she caused the patient, and her failure to report the incident, Mary faces an action against her for malpractice, termination, public reprimand, censure, loss of certification, and loss of license. She will most likely find herself defending her actions before the ethics body of her professional association, her professional certification board, and her state's licensure board.

One's choices do not end with the law. Sometimes a more compelling social reason exists to cause one to stray from what some consider the letter of the law. For example, one might justify breaking the law against speeding to deliver a sick child to the hospital as quickly as possible. When presented with the choice to drive the speed limit and risk the child's life versus driving above the speed limit to give the child a fighting chance of survival, one might choose to break the law.

On the other hand, one may face two good choices. However, certain other laws may present choices that, although not equally good, tip the scales in one direction or the other based on one's value system. It is important to identify all the angles.

One must not ignore the law, the social consequences, or one's own moral suppositions. In some situations, the social consequences may dictate choices, whereas in others the law compels action.

This does not mean one should act outside the law, one's professional code of ethics, or one's personal value system. However, black and white answers do not always present themselves. One must weigh the alternatives and make choices. At the same time, one must not limit one's view of a particular situation to the legal perspective, one's personal values, or one's code of ethics. One must consider all perspectives, balance them, and make choices.

REFERENCE

Seldes, G. (1972). *The great quotations.* New York: Simon & Schuster.

6

Analyzing Ethical Dilemmas

"The mass of men lead lives of quiet desperation."
Henry David Thoreau, quoted in Baker, 1992

So you have identified an ethical dilemma. Perhaps this dilemma causes you to feel that familiar discomfort in your gut. What happens next?

To respond properly when faced with an ethical dilemma, one must do more than simply react. Every health professional serves many masters: one's self, the patient, one's employer, the law, and one's profession, to name a few. How do professionals balance these often conflicting demands? Ethical decision making requires effort. With training, self-reflection, and practice, one's ability to resolve ethical dilemmas can effectively improve.

The analysis of any ethical dilemma involves a multistep process and, as we have seen, many different sets of values are available to serve as guides. No absolutely right or wrong way exists to analyze an ethical issue. What is important is that some analysis takes place.

Several methods or processing tools exist to analyze ethical dilemmas (Jonsen, Seigler, & Winslade, 1998; Purtillo, 1993; Trompetter, Hansen, & Kyler-Hutchison, 1998). The authors propose a framework for analysis—one approach to learning the ethical decision-making process. It requires a comprehensive analysis of many factors as a means of preparing the professional or student to make well-reasoned ethical choices.

The method of analyzing ethical dilemmas presented by the authors considers both legal and ethical issues. The CELIBATE method (Clinical Ethics & Legal Issues Bait All Therapists Equally) (Table 6-1) for analyzing ethical dilemmas, developed by the authors, gives readers a framework for analyzing ethical dilemmas typically occurring in therapy practice. This method considers legal issues and accepts legal issues as an integral part of looking at ethical dilemmas. Section II, the ethical dilemma workbook section, presents readers with 115 ethical dilemmas from actual practice and educational situations. Readers can practice the CELIBATE method using the dilemmas found in this section of the book.

To illustrate use of the CELIBATE method, the authors present the following case study:

CASE STUDY

Mary, a fieldwork student at the Really Really Rehab Center, has struggled throughout her affiliation. Calling her performance marginal would be a compliment. As her supervisor, you have repeatedly given her specific feedback, instructing her in ways to change her behavior. Unfortunately, Mary fails to heed any of your advice. At midterm, Mary's performance merited a failing grade. Mary forgets to lock the brakes on wheelchairs and shows a disregard for many other safety precautions.

Table 6-1

CELIBATE Method for Analyzing Ethical Dilemmas
(Clinical Ethics and Legal Issues Bait All Therapists Equally)

1. What is the problem?
2. What are the facts of the situation?
3. Who are the interested parties?
   - Facility, patient, other therapists, observers, payers, etc.
4. What is the nature of the interest? Why is this a problem?
   - Professional
   - Personal
   - Business
   - Economic
   - Intellectual
   - Societal
5. Ethical?
   - Does it violate a professional code of ethics?
   - Which section(s)?
6. Legal? Is there a legal issue?
   - Practice act/licensure law and regulations?
   - Other laws: Check the CELIBATE checklist
7. Do I need more information?
   - What information do I need?
   - Is there a treatment, policy, procedure, law, regulation, or document that I do not know about?
   - Can I obtain a copy of the treatment, policy, procedure, law, regulation, or document in writing?
   - Do I need to research the issue further?
   - Do I need to consult with a mentor, an expert in this area, or a lawyer?
8. Brainstorm possible action steps
9. Analyze action steps
   - Eliminate obvious wrong or impossible choices
   - How will each alternative affect my patients, other interested parties, and me?
   - Do my choices abide by the code of ethics?
   - Do my choices abide by the practice act and regulations?
   - Are my choices consistent with my moral, religious, and social beliefs?
10. Choose a course of action
    - The Rotary four-way test
      Is it the truth?
      Is it fair to all concerned?
      Will it build goodwill and better friendships?
      Will it be beneficial to all concerned?
    - Is it win-win?
    - How do I feel about my course of action?

You now approach the final evaluation. After spending a half hour struggling with this failing final evaluation, the rehabilitation director, looking over your shoulder, tells you not to fail Mary because Mary has done her best despite a learning disability. "Even though she really failed this fieldwork, it's just too much trouble to give her a failing grade," the rehabilitation director tells you. The rehabilitation director also reminds you that the hospital does not want to be sued for an ADA (Americans with Disabilities Act) violation should Mary fail her fieldwork. You had no previous knowledge of Mary's learning disability—only of her failing performance.

WHAT IS THE PROBLEM?

Before one can begin to analyze an ethical dilemma, one must identify the problem. The first step in the analysis identifies the problem and sets the stage for the remaining analysis. What is the problem in the case study? The rehabilitation director wants the supervisor to pass a fieldwork student whose failing performance does not warrant a passing grade. This situation would probably cause most supervisors some inner conflict and discomfort. Thoughts such as, "How can I pass a student whose performance fails to measure to a passing level?" or "Is passing this student the right thing to do?" would probably travel through a supervisor's mind. Does passing Mary comport with the ethical principle of justice? Autonomy? Paternalism?

WHAT ARE THE FACTS OF THE SITUATION?

"To solve a problem it is necessary to think. It is necessary to think even to decide what facts to collect."
Robert Maynard Hutchins, quoted in Peter, 1977

After identifying the problem, the next step takes readers to the facts of the situation. Here, one must identify all the facts. The facts help determine the interests of the parties involved and help narrow down action steps.

Looking at the case study, one can identity the following facts:

- ◆ Mary works as a fieldwork student at Really Really Rehab Center
- ◆ Her performance at midterm equaled a failing grade
- ◆ Mary's supervisor provided her with adequate supervision, including specific feedback regarding ways to improve her behavior
- ◆ Mary failed to modify her behavior in response to the supervisor's feedback
- ◆ Mary forgets to abide by many patient safety precautions and, in particular, fails to lock wheelchair brakes
- ◆ Mary's performance at the end of her fieldwork continues to warrant a failing grade
- ◆ The supervisor feels Mary earned a failing grade and she planned to fail her
- ◆ The rehabilitation director instructs the supervisor not to fail Mary
- ◆ At the end of the fieldwork, the rehabilitation director informs the supervisor for the first time that Mary has a learning disability
- ◆ In assigning Mary a failing grade, the supervisor did not consider Mary's disability
- ◆ The rehabilitation director tells the supervisor

not to fail Mary because she fears the hospital will face a lawsuit under the ADA

WHO ARE THE INTERESTED PARTIES?

This step considers all the parties who may have an interest in the ethical dilemma, either because the outcome will directly or indirectly affect them or because it has the potential to directly or indirectly affect them.

WHAT IS THE NATURE OF THE INTEREST? WHY IS THIS A PROBLEM?

- ◆ Professional
- ◆ Personal
- ◆ Business
- ◆ Economic
- ◆ Intellectual
- ◆ Societal

In this step, we look at the interested parties and identify their interests. Table 6-2 identifies the interested parties in the case study and displays their interests side by side.

IS THERE AN ETHICAL ISSUE?

Does it Violate a Professional Code of Ethics? Which Section(s)?

This inquiry requires readers to carefully review their own professional code of ethics and compare the action to the code. In the case study, passing a student who earns a failing grade at the very least violates code of ethics provisions addressing justice, veracity, and probably nonmaleficence, because the student will likely harm someone in the future.

Does it Violate Moral, Social, or Religious Values?

This inquiry looks into oneself to one's own personal set of moral, social, and religious values. In this case study, the supervisor may find that failing

Table 6-2

Interested Parties and Their Interests

INTERESTED PARTIES	THEIR INTERESTS
Mary	Personal—needs a job, needs to pass, does not want the embarrassment of failure Professional—wants a license, desires to practice Economic—wants to work
Mary's parents, who paid for her education	Economic—do not want to waste their money Personal—embarrassment, hurt because their daughter failed
The supervisor	Professional—wants competent therapists; wants her professional reputation intact Personal—wants her personal reputation intact and does not want a failing student to pass Business—must balance management's need with duty to patients and their safety
The rehabilitation director	Business—wants to avoid litigation Economic—wants to avoid the costs of litigation
Really Really Rehab Center	Same as rehabilitation director Business—wants to maintain its reputation in the community
Mary's future potential patients	Personal—need safe and competent care
Mary's future employers	Business—need to hire competent therapists and avoid litigation
The federal government	Societal—wants to ensure that individuals with a disability are not denied opportunity
Academic program from which Mary came	Business—wants to uphold reputation Economic—wants to keep students in the program Professional—abiding interest in the competency of the graduates of the program
Other therapists at the Really Really Rehab Center	Economic—do not want anything to compromise the economic health of the facility Professional—desire the facility to maintain its reputation because their individual reputation depends on it Personal—do not want to see a failing student pass
Other fieldwork students at Really Really Rehab Center	Professional—do not want their reputations tarnished because a failing student was given a passing grade Personal—resentment at the incompetent student receiving a passing grade
The ADA coordinator at the Really Really Rehab Center	Professional—desires to avoid ADA litigation Economic—desires to avoid ADA litigation and keep her job
Liability insurance carriers (companies) for both the academic program and the Really Really Rehab Center	Economic—desire to not pay out claims for malpractice
Mary's professional association	Professional—wants to maintain standards of competency and ethics Societal—wants to maintain standards of competency and ethics
State licensing board	Professional—wants to protect citizenry by maintaining standards of competency and ethics Societal—wants to protect citizenry by maintaining standards of competency and ethics

Mary is tantamount to lying, which violates her moral and religious beliefs. These personal beliefs make this a more difficult decision for the supervisor than for others who may not share her religious or moral beliefs.

IS THERE A LEGAL ISSUE?

Practice Act/Licensure Law and Regulations?

At this point in the analysis, readers must review their own practice acts/licensure laws as well as the regulations. This will help readers determine whether passing Mary violates the licensure law and its regulations. Appendix B contains sample practice acts. In Florida, for example, the Occupational Therapy Practice Act prohibits the filing of false documents. Should the supervisor pass Mary, this action might violate this provision of Florida's Practice Act and regulations because the evaluation would contain false information.

Other Laws: Check the CELIBATE Checklist

A review of the CELIBATE checklist (Table 6-3) gives the reader information about common legal problems that may arise in ethical dilemmas in practice and education. This list does not include every legal issue that may arise—only those the authors have noted to arise most commonly. The legal issues marked with an asterisk may fall into the criminal as well as civil law categories. This means one may find oneself criminally liable if involved in those offenses.

Readers will find that the CELIBATE checklist helps to narrow down choices of action. Readers can identify legal issues that may point toward or away from specific choices. As the name implies, readers will want to stay away from the legal issues identified on the CELIBATE checklist to avoid civil, as well as criminal, liability.

In the case study, we find several possible legal issues. These include the following:

- ◆ ADA
- ◆ Filing a false report

- ◆ Practice act/licensure law (violating the code of ethics and/or failing to report an ethical violation)
- ◆ Negligent supervision (of the student should she harm a patient in the future)
- ◆ Breach of contract (between the school and the facility)
- ◆ Confidentiality of student records (How did the rehabilitation director find out about Mary's disability? Did she call the school for information?)

DO I NEED MORE INFORMATION?

At this point, readers may have questions for which they need answers. However, the questions may require additional concrete information, such as patient records, policies and procedures, or other documents to obtain answers.

What Information Do I Need?

A range of information might help in this situation. For example, the supervisor might want to know whether this is the student's last fieldwork placement. If the student will do another fieldwork assignment, the supervisor might count on the next supervisor to fail Mary.

Is There a Treatment, Policy, Procedure, Law, Regulation, or Document That I Do Not Know About?

The supervisor might want to familiarize herself with the ADA.

Can I Obtain a Copy of the Treatment, Policy, Procedure, Law, Regulation, or Document in Writing?

In the case study, the supervisor can obtain the applicable ADA regulations online, download them, and read them. In some situations where policy matters come into question, facilities may not have a written policy or may not provide a copy.

Table 6-3

CELIBATE Checklist
(Clinical Ethics and Legal Issues Bait All Therapists Equally)

Is there a legal issue?	Yes	No
Age discrimination?		
Antitrust?		
Assault and/or battery?*		
Breach of contract?		
Child abuse?*		
Copyright violations?*		
Confidentiality of student records?		
Covenants not to compete?		
Disability discrimination?		
Elder abuse?*		
Embezzlement?*		
Employee/independent contractor?		
Family Medical Leave Act?		
Fraud? (Insurance)*		
Gag clauses?		
Guardianship/conservatorship?		
Kickbacks?*		
Malpractice?		
Medicare fraud?*		
Modalities without training?		
Negligence?		
OBRA violation?		
Patient confidentiality?		
Plagiarism?		
Sex discrimination?		
Sex with a patient?*		
Sexual harassment?		
Spousal abuse?*		
Theft?*		
Trade secrets?		
Treatment without a prescription or referral?*		
Violation of privacy laws? (AIDS in Florida)*		

*May fall into criminal as well as civil law categories

Do I Need to Research the Issue Further?

The supervisor may wish to seek other resources to find more information about the issue.

Do I Need to Consult With a Mentor, an Expert in This Area, or a Lawyer?

The supervisor may want to contact another clinical fieldwork coordinator from another facility or someone who deals with fieldwork issues at her professional association for assistance. Mentors provide invaluable assistance in these situations, allowing you to process your ideas and receive feedback. In this situation, the supervisor probably would not seek a lawyer's advice. However, lawyers can provide necessary advice, for example, in dealing with contract issues and suspected fraudulent practices. In some situations, consulting a lawyer can keep readers away from potential liability—both civil and criminal.

BRAINSTORM POSSIBLE ACTION STEPS

"To understand is hard. Once one understands, action is easy."
Sun Yat-Sen, quoted in Seldes, 1972

This step takes the reader on a journey of creative thought and self-exploration. In this step, readers synthesize the facts of the dilemma with their own beliefs to articulate a range of possible action steps. By the nature of the process, some action steps bring more appeal to the table than do others. The goal is to articulate as many action steps as possible, so the element of choice remains vibrant.

In the case study, some of the choices the supervisor might consider include:

- Fail Mary
- Pass Mary
- Call the academic program and ask the academic fieldwork coordinator what to do
- Research the ADA as to whether she can give Mary a failing grade for failing performance
- Visit the ADA coordinator for the hospital and get more information
- Complain to the rehabilitation director's immediate supervisor
- Call the police
- Call Mary's parents
- Contact the justice department that enforces the ADA and ask them if failing Mary violates the ADA
- Consult with an ADA lawyer
- Discuss the situation with her spouse
- Discuss the situation with her religious or spiritual advisor for advice
- Quit the job rather than pass Mary

ANALYZE ACTION STEPS

"Think like a man of action, act like a man of thought."
Henri Bergson, quoted in Peter, 1977

In this step, readers critically review the action steps brainstormed in the previous step to narrow down the choices.

Eliminate Obvious Wrong or Impossible Choices

In the case study, several choices would fall by the wayside as obviously wrong or impossible choices. For example, calling the police accomplishes nothing. This matter falls outside police jurisdiction and concern as it does not involve a criminal issue the police enforce. Contacting Mary's parents would also not help the situation and would probably inappropriately violate confidentiality.

How Will Each Alternative Affect My Patients, Other Interested Parties, and Me?

The reader may wish to explore how his or her decision will impact these parties.

Do My Choices Abide by the Applicable Code of Ethics?

The reader may want to revisit the code of ethics of his or her profession.

Do My Choices Abide by the Applicable Practice Act and Regulations?

The reader may want to familiarize himself or herself with the state's practice act and regulations.

Are My Choices Consistent With My Moral, Religious, and Social Beliefs?

After discarding the obviously incorrect choices, readers complete their analysis of the specific choices, looking first at how each choice affects patients and other interested parties. The field of choice narrows down as readers compare their remaining possible actions with the requirements of their code of ethics and practice act and regulations. The final analysis looks to oneself to compare possible choices with one's moral, religious, and social beliefs.

CHOOSE A COURSE OF ACTION

Once readers choose a course of action, they can analyze an action step in several ways. Rotary International, a large service organization, encourages its members to evaluate "the things they say or do" using the four-way test (Taylor, 1932). Readers will find answering the questions in the Rotary four-way test helpful in analyzing their own behavior.

The Rotary Four-Way Test

1. Is it the truth?
2. Is it fair to all concerned?
3. Will it build goodwill and better friendships?
4. Will it be beneficial to all concerned?

Is It Win-Win?

Readers can consider whether the action sets up a win-win situation, which is the most just result for any ethical dilemma.

How Do You Feel About Your Course of Action?

Finally, readers can evaluate their actions by analyzing a visceral response. How do you feel about your course of action?

With this information in hand, readers can practice what they have learned by tackling the ethical dilemmas in Section II.

REFERENCES

Baker, D. B. (1992). *Power quotes.* Detroit, MI: Visible Ink Press.

Jonsen, A. R., Seigler, M., & Winslade, W. J. (1998). *Clinical ethics.* New York: McGraw Hill.

Peter, L. J. (1977). *Peter's quotations.* New York: Quill, William Morrow.

Purtillo, R. (1993). *Ethical dimensions in the health professions.* Philadelphia, PA: W. B. Saunders.

Seldes, G. (1972). *The great quotations.* New York: Simon & Schuster.

Taylor, H. (1932). *The four-way test.* Available http://www.rotary.org/whatis/part_II.htm#4way.

Trompetter, L., Hansen, R., & Kyler-Hutchison, P. (1998). *Reference guide to the occupational therapy code of ethics.* Bethesda, MD: American Occupational Therapy Association.

7

Avoiding Ethical and Legal Dilemmas

With all the potential pitfalls in health care today, how can we protect ourselves from falling victim to legal and ethical problems? Just remember to "protect thy patients & thyself" (Table 7-1).

PUT A COPY OF YOUR LICENSURE LAW ON YOUR DESK AND READ IT

This painless step can prove invaluable for practitioners. Many of us have never seen our own licensure law, let alone taken the time to read it. Read it and digest it.

Once you finish reading the licensure law, do not file it away. Keep it on your desk so you can refer to it often. Make a note in your calendar to read it again in a month or two, and a month or two after that. Take the time to find out when those in charge update your licensure law, and while you are at it, drop by a meeting of your state licensure board. You might learn something new that can help you protect yourself and your patients.

REPORT ETHICAL AND LEGAL VIOLATIONS TO ETHICS AND LICENSURE BOARDS

Most professional codes of ethics require those subject to the code to report known violations by others. Most licensure boards also impose the duty to report those in violation of the licensure law. Do not look at reporting as "tattling"; look at it as maintaining the integrity of your profession. It is your ethical obligation.

OPEN YOUR EYES

If something does not seem right, it probably is not. Sometimes in practice supervisors and administrators tell us to do things that just do not seem right. Consequences arise that we do not anticipate. Do not follow blindly. Your gut reaction probably has some merit. Look into it further.

	Table 7-1	
	Protect Thy Patients & Thyself	
P	Put a copy of your licensure law on your desk and read it	
R	Report ethical violations to ethics and licensure boards	
O	Open your eyes	
T	Tell them you want it in writing	
E	Encourage ethical behavior	
C	Cover yourself with contemporaneous, complete, and comprehensive documentation—evaluations and progress notes ("The 4 C's")	
T	Think	
T	Take the patient's interest above all	
H	Handle situations as they arise	
Y	Yearn to learn	
P	Plug into your professional associations	
A	Ask a lot of questions if you are unsure of an action or task someone wants you to perform	
T	Train and supervise all subordinates properly	
I	Invest in a newspaper subscription	
E	Establish a relationship with a mentor	
N	Never fall behind	
T	Take a good look at the professional literature	
S	Surf the Internet for changes in regulations under which you work	
&		
T	Take the time to read your professional code of ethics and standards of practice	
H	Hand over patients to those with more expertise	
Y	Yield to the dictates of Medicare regulations and other rules and regulations with which you work on a regular basis	
S	Save a copy of all written correspondence	
E	Explore all alternatives	
L	Look at professional association home pages on a regular basis for changes	
F	Fill out all forms accurately and truthfully	

TELL THEM YOU WANT IT IN WRITING

If something does not make sense to you, or you find yourself questioning an order, get it in writing. The person requesting the action will probably not put the requested illegal action in writing. The same may hold true with requests for unethical behaviors. However, supervisors and administrators may not understand the ethical consequences of an action, especially if they do not share the same professional code of ethics. Above all, they may not care about your ethics.

Requesting instruction in writing works well with requests for changing documentation or billing after the fact. Often the instructions change after the therapist requests the order in writing. If you do obtain the request in writing, you will create a paper trail of the request and your subsequent actions. In another variation of this same technique, you write your own memo to the person who requested the action, stating your understanding of the request and asking for written verification. Alternatively, you can ask for a copy of the written policy.

ENCOURAGE ETHICAL BEHAVIOR

Encourage colleagues to read their code of ethics. Read and study the code together in a group. Organize informal discussion groups about ethical issues. Review the ethical dilemmas from this book in a group and process responses with each other at work. Post an ethical principle of the week in the classroom or clinic. Make ethics the topic of inservice training in your setting. Make ethics a priority. Let everyone know you believe ethical behavior is important.

Cover Yourself With Contemporaneous, Complete, and Comprehensive Documentation—Evaluations and Progress Notes ("The 4 C's")

Keep in mind that documentation probably plays the most significant role in protecting yourself and your patients. Document as close to the treatment session as possible so your progress notes do not become a work of fiction. Make sure notes are complete, discussing the type of treatment the patient underwent and the patient's response in functional terms. Do not change documentation after the fact and do not allow others to influence you to change your documentation or to include untruths or misstatements.

Think

It is amazing how many students and therapists panic first and think later. You have many answers inside you if you just take the time to think. While you are thinking, consider purchasing malpractice insurance.

Take the Patient's Interest Above All

Using this philosophy, you should find yourself safe from ethical problems. Some therapists report leaving a job over unethical behavior in which they refused to participate, choosing instead to protect the patient and quit. Obviously, this choice did not come easily.

Handle Situations as They Arise

Do not let problem situations fester. As time goes by, you will find that solutions and choices are more difficult than at the problem's inception. Treating people nicely also makes for fewer problems. Physicians known for their good bedside manner find themselves facing fewer malpractice actions.

Yearn to Learn

Take advantage of all continuing education opportunities. Learning continues past the university walls. Should you find yourself facing a malpractice action, another therapist will testify to the accepted professional standard expected of you. The professional standard includes your level of knowledge about your area of specialty or focus. You must continuously learn about your area of specialty. Professional codes of ethics encourage continuing education. Continuing education opportunities constantly expand, especially with Internet access. Many professional associations and educational institutions provide courses online and online access expands daily.

Plug Into Your Professional Associations/Join Your State and National Associations

Both types of organizations can provide you with valuable information about practice, education, and the status of changing laws and regulations, which you must follow.

State and national organizations often associate with lobbyists who work to support legislative efforts to benefit the profession. Often these lobbying efforts act as "preventative medicine" to avoid legislation that is not in the profession's or patient's best interest.

Ask a Lot of Questions If You Are Unsure of an Action or Task Someone Would Like You to Perform

Ask questions until you feel satisfied with the answer. If you do not ask questions, you may end up doing something illegal or unethical.

Some people fear that they appear unintelligent when they ask questions. By asking questions before acting, however, therapists can learn crucial information to assist them in making both ethical and legal choices. For example, when asked to perform an unfamiliar treatment for the first time, students and new therapists will probably need to ask questions about the treatment procedures. Asking questions about uncertain actions can protect both the therapist and the patient. Better to look dim-witted than to harm a patient.

Properly Train and Supervise All Subordinates

Legally, you are responsible for the actions of your subordinates. You may find yourself facing a malpractice act for their negligent actions.

Do not delegate activities to subordinates for which they lack adequate training. Do not delegate responsibilities or tasks to subordinates that violate licensure laws or regulations. Take care to not let the pressure for productivity influence your judgment and compromise your ethics.

Invest in a Newspaper Subscription

The newspaper provides invaluable information about proposed changes to laws and regulations. The newspaper also notifies you when laws affecting Medicare, IDEA (Individuals with Disabilities Educational Act), and similar institutions change. Newspaper subscriptions cost very little and provide much information for rehabilitation professionals. Staying on top of the news is one way to protect your patients and yourself. Most major newspapers provide major stories on the Internet. See the Internet resources contained in Appendix R for newspaper websites.

Establish a Relationship With a Mentor

Mentors can provide invaluable advice and support. Sometimes just bouncing ideas off a mentor can help clarify one's actions. The mentor may provide additional information or a different perspective on a situation. Further, mentors can help by raising questions and issues not yet considered.

Never Fall Behind

Keep all paperwork and documentation up to date. This tidbit of seemingly obvious advice protects both the patient and the therapist and comports with both ethical and legal demands.

Take a Look at the Professional Literature

Read your professional literature. It helps create the standard of care for your profession—the standard to which you must practice. Although not every article in your professional literature will apply to your practice, you must read and adjust your practice to the ones that do.

Surf the Internet for Changes in Regulations Under Which You Work

The Internet provides nearly instantaneous information about regulations as they change. Therapists can surf the web and find entire regulations online. Increasingly, we see states putting their laws and regulations and proposed laws and regulations online. Therapists can also locate a wealth of information about ethics online. See Appendix R for Internet resources for helpful legal and ethics sites.

TAKE THE TIME TO READ YOUR PROFESSIONAL CODE OF ETHICS AND STANDARDS OF PRACTICE

Understand your responsibilities under each one. Keep them handy and read them often. Most professional associations make their codes of ethics available online.

HAND OVER PATIENTS TO THOSE WITH MORE EXPERTISE

Not all therapists are equal. At some time during your career, you may encounter a situation with which you lack familiarity or experience. When appropriate, refer patients to professionals who are better equipped to treat the patient's particular problem.

YIELD TO THE DICTATES OF MEDICARE REGULATIONS AND OTHER RULES AND REGULATIONS WITH WHICH YOU WORK ON A REGULAR BASIS

You work under a set of rules that govern your behavior. No one expects you to become an attorney, but you are responsible for your behavior and that behavior can get you in trouble if you do not know the rules. You need to understand the Medicare regulations and other rules and regulations with which you work to assure your compliance with their mandates. Although some say ignorance is bliss, reality reminds us that ignorance of the law is no excuse.

SAVE A COPY OF ALL WRITTEN CORRESPONDENCE

This creates a paper trail in case you need it later to document your actions to a licensure or ethics board.

EXPLORE ALL ALTERNATIVES

Use the CELIBATE method for analyzing ethical dilemmas to look at all perspectives of a situation before you act.

LOOK AT PROFESSIONAL ASSOCIATION HOME PAGES ON A REGULAR BASIS FOR CHANGES

Most home pages contain information about the latest changes affecting the profession. Most webpages link to sites of interest to the profession. For example, the American Occupational Therapy Association site (www.aota.org) is linked to a wealth of information about the prospective payment system both before and after the government announced its adoption. The American Speech-Language Hearing Association (www.asha.org) linked its homepage to the IDEA Part B regulations almost contemporaneously with the government's announcing their release.

FILL OUT ALL FORMS ACCURATELY AND TRUTHFULLY

Resist temptations and pressures to exaggerate or falsely report information on forms required by the government and insurance payers.

CONCLUSION

Therapists can take many steps to avoid legal and ethical problems in practice. However, no one can insulate himself or herself from the realities of rehabilitation practice today. Ultimately, those realities continue to present clinicians with situations that require one to make choices.

SECTION
II

Ethical Dilemmas: Practical Applications

Dilemma 1: *You are a home health therapist. Another therapist asks you to cover her caseload while she is on vacation. After you have seen all of the therapist's patients once, you realize that they are all functioning well and really no longer need therapy.*

Dilemma 2: *You are treating a patient in home health care who has a fractured pelvis from a car accident. As a result of your excellent intervention, the patient becomes independent in all functional skills. The patient looks disappointed and tells you, "My lawyer said this is bad for my case. I need to complain more." In response to your questions the patient tells you, "My lawyer said if I don't have a permanent disability I will lose my case."*

Dilemma 3: *A few of the therapists in your department treat home health patients after work hours for a private home health agency. On several occasions, you have seen the therapists taking home bandages and other supplies, which they never return.*

Dilemma 4: *You are treating a patient under workers' compensation. Certain billing codes are reimbursed at higher rates than others. Your patient has trouble dressing himself because of bilateral shoulder fractures. You find the actual treatment you are providing is not reimbursed well. In fact, the treatment is reimbursed at the lowest rate. You could bill for this patient under the code for another type of treatment, which is reimbursed at the highest rate.*

Dilemma 5: *You are a home health therapist. Most of the patients you treat are through Medicare home health agencies. You get a call from another home health therapist who refers a patient to you because the therapist is moving out of town. The patient is a "private pay" patient. The patient, Mrs. Brown, will pay you cash for each treatment. You thank the other therapist for the referral and ask her for her notes. She replies, "I don't have notes. The patient is private pay and you do not need them for reimbursement."*

Dilemma 6: *Mrs. Johnson is referred to therapy for treatment. She is 86 years old and has made it very clear to you that she is waiting to die and does not want any therapy.*

Dilemma 7: *You are asked to do some staff training at a local nursing home. When you arrive you discover the activities room has a large sign on it that reads "Therapy." None of the staff members in the "therapy" department are trained therapists or certified/licensed therapy assistants.*

See Pages 93-110 for Ethical Dilemma Worksheets

Dilemma 8: *During the social hour at a meeting of local therapists in private practice, a discussion comes up about fees. All of the therapists agree that they are not charging their HMO enough for their services. The therapists agree that each member of the group will charge the same higher fee for therapy services.*

Dilemma 9: *You are a certified/licensed therapy assistant in a pediatric clinic. You notice that every Monday morning, Billy, a 5-year-old patient, comes to therapy with bruises all over his body and small round marks that look a lot like cigarette burns on his legs. When you ask Billy about the bruises outside the presence of his mother, he stutters and replies, "I fall a lot."*

Dilemma 10: *Your facility has a skeleton staff on Saturdays. Because of the limited staff, the policy states that you see only patients on the rehabilitation floor on Saturdays as a priority, as the reimbursement is higher and, for now, DRG exempt. According to the policy, acute care patients from the rest of the hospital are not seen on Saturdays. You are working on Saturday and receive a STAT order for treatment of a 67-year-old woman who had emergency surgery. You also receive an order to evaluate a new acute care patient with a stroke.*

Dilemma 11: *You are working on an inpatient psychiatric ward of a teaching hospital. Mrs. Denton is admitted with a diagnosis of "hysterical stroke." You evaluate her and find that among other things, she has slurred speech, difficulty swallowing, and she drools out of one side of her mouth. In fact, you think Mrs. Denton may be aspirating her food. Based on the results of your evaluation, you believe that Mrs. Denton has had a real stroke, and you believe the care she is getting in the psychiatric unit is not appropriate for someone who just had a CVA.*

Dilemma 12: *You are the director of a therapy department. The director of rehabilitation has given you a lot of negative feedback lately at department head meetings because the statistics of other therapy departments have been much higher than your department's statistics. While routinely reviewing some medical and department records, you discover positive proof that the director of the other therapy department has been exaggerating patient statistics to reflect a greater patient-to-therapist ratio than actually exists.*

Dilemma 13: *You work inhouse for an HMO. Company policy allows you to see patients two times per week for 1 hour each time for a maximum of 4 weeks. You are instructed that at the end of the 4 weeks you must write a note for each patient stating the patient no longer needs therapy services. Henry, a 30-year-old man who is developmentally disabled with an IQ of 60, is referred to therapy by a hand surgeon. While leaning on a window, Henry accidentally put his hand through the glass, severing the median and ulna nerves and several extensor and flexor tendons. Following the surgical repair of the many severed tendons, Henry is referred to therapy by his hand surgeon with an order that states "therapy 5x per week for 2 months and return to MD for further orders."*

See Pages 93-110 for Ethical Dilemma Worksheets

Dilemma 14: *You have been trying to treat Mrs. Rodriguez for 2 weeks. Mrs. Rodriguez is an 86-year-old woman who does not want therapy (although she needs it). She insists she does not need to learn what you are trying to teach her because in her culture, that is what family is for—to take care of you when you get old. After trying everything to convince Mrs. Rodriguez to participate in therapy, you finally discharge her. Mrs. Rodriguez's daughter comes to see you to complain about how you inappropriately discharged her mother.*

Dilemma 15: *Mr. Robinson is very weak and can only tolerate a 10-minute treatment session. You are hoping to build up his tolerance. You treat him for 10 minutes per the doctor's order. However, your treatment facility bills therapy in 15-minute units.*

Dilemma 16: *The contract company you work for has decided to save money by eliminating the patient transporters. Under the new policy, therapists are to transport patients to therapy themselves and bill every patient one unit (a unit being equal to 15 minutes) for an activity of daily living—mobility independence training. Sally Fitzpatrick is a 25-year-old woman recovering from a traumatic brain injury. She is at Ranchos Los Amigos level 3. Mobility independence training is not a realistic treatment for her at this point in her coma recovery. You do not feel it is right to bill Sally for treatment you are not providing but you know your billing is reviewed for the daily "transport" unit.*

Dilemma 17: *The company you work for is trying a new approach for increasing productivity. For every unit you bill over a set amount, you get points credited toward a trip to Disney World. You have always wanted to go to Disney World.*

Dilemma 18: *You have decided to return to school part-time to advance your training in your professional discipline. You realize very quickly the price of textbooks has significantly increased since you completed your last level of training. Two other part-time students in the class approach you about pooling resources and buying one set of books to share. Because each of you has access to a copy machine at work, they suggest purchasing one of each textbook for the group and having each person make two copies of one of the books so each person gets a copy of each textbook.*

Dilemma 19: *You are a therapist in a rural school district where there are no therapists of other disciplines. The district has been unable to get therapists from other disciplines despite numerous recruiting efforts and a current open position. Jennie, a kindergarten student, has mild cerebral palsy. She is bright but not yet walking, her language is delayed, and she is unable to perform ADLs as expected for her age. During an IEP (individualized education plan), both parents and teacher request you focus more on teaching skills generally addressed by another discipline and less on skills generally addressed by your discipline. You are not comfortable teaching this child.*

See Pages 93-110 for Ethical Dilemma Worksheets

Dilemma 20: *Like many other facilities, your hospital has decided to reorganize. You have been appointed to head up the head injury team. This means you now supervise therapists in several disciplines working with patients recovering from traumatic brain injuries. Among other things, you will be responsible for conducting performance appraisals. You are not sure you understand the role of two of the disciplines under your supervision.*

Dilemma 21: *You work in an inpatient psychiatric unit. Dr. Billings has referred a new patient to you, Carol, who has a diagnosis of anxiety disorder and depression with a history of suicidal ideation. You have worked with the patient for three treatment sessions. Carol has orders to participate in the field trip scheduled for the afternoon, and you will be one of the therapists accompanying the patients. Based on your treatment sessions with Carol, you do not feel it is wise for her to go off the hospital grounds at this time. She has told you several times that she has dreams about running out in front of oncoming traffic and the pleasant feeling she felt floating up to heaven. You have recorded this in your progress notes. You call Dr. Billings' office and after you share your concerns with him, he tells you he wants Carol to go on the field trip anyway. You still do not feel comfortable taking Carol out.*

Dilemma 22: *Your hospital has a new policy. You may treat private-pay patients for up to 2 hours per day, which is no change from the previous policy. However, Medicaid patients may only be seen for a maximum of two units per day (15 minutes equals one unit). Ken is a 36-year-old Medicaid patient with a recent CVA. He has excellent therapeutic potential and good endurance. You feel he will benefit from the 2 hours per day of treatment non-Medicaid patients receive.*

Dilemma 23: *You are supervising Diana, a fieldwork student in the hospital where you work. You are assigned to work with a new patient who you immediately assign to Diana. The patient, Jack Harper, is a 40-year-old television news reporter for the major network affiliate in your town. While reading the chart, your student discovers Mr. Harper has AIDS. Although she has not yet told anyone at the fieldwork site, she now tells you she is 8 weeks pregnant and she does not want to treat Mr. Harper because of her pregnancy.*

Dilemma 24: *You are assigned to treat Jack Harper, a 40-year-old television news reporter for the major network affiliate in your town. While reading the chart, you discover he has AIDS. Although you have not yet told anyone at work, you are 8 weeks pregnant and you really do not want to treat Mr. Harper.*

Dilemma 25: *You are assigned to treat Jack Harper, a 40-year-old television news reporter for the major network affiliate in your town and local celebrity. While reading the chart, you discover he has AIDS. Later that evening at dinner, you mention to your spouse that Jack Harper is your new patient. Your spouse asks you what Harper "is in for." In the past you have discussed this sort of information about nameless patients with your spouse.*

See Pages 93-110 for Ethical Dilemma Worksheets

Dilemma 26: *You are very busy at work so you decide to catch up on some of your work by bringing patients' therapy charts home so you can write your notes. You work at the kitchen table after dinner. You return from a bathroom break to find your teenage son reading through one of your patient's charts. You live in a small community where everyone knows everyone else—and their business.*

Dilemma 27: *You work for a therapy company that contracts with long-term health care facilities. Your company has just obtained a contract with the nursing home to which you have been assigned. After about a month of working there, you realize that all of the patients seen by therapy are restrained with vest-type restraints, commonly referred to as posey restraints. Because you do not work directly for the nursing home, you do not feel comfortable saying anything, although on several occasions, you have tactfully dropped hints about this issue—to no avail. You decide to complain to the therapy company but your supervisor tells you not to worry about the restraints and to "stay out of this one" because it has nothing to do with your ability to provide therapy to the patients.*

Dilemma 28: *You work in a psychiatric hospital. You and your coworkers decide to go to a local bar for happy hour after work. Penny and Bob begin to joke about Mrs. Nixon's delusional system and some of the amusing things she did this week. Betty jumps in with Mr. Yamamoto's antics in the psychiatric unit. Several others join in this rather loud conversation about patients.*

Dilemma 29: *You work in a large therapy department in a large hospital. You find out that therapists in another discipline are being paid higher salaries than the therapists in your discipline, even though the billing rates and charges for both therapy services are the same.*

Dilemma 30: *Your state has recently instituted a continuing education requirement for licensure renewal. You attend two continuing education workshops with a rather large attendance at each one. Several of your coworkers are also attending these workshops. At each workshop, after about 1 hour, one of your coworkers leaves the workshop. Approximately 1 hour before the program is scheduled to end, your coworker returns with several overstuffed shopping bags from the mall, just in time to receive her certificate of attendance indicating she attended the full 6.5 hours.*

Dilemma 31: *You attend an important regional therapy conference. You decide to show support for Laura, a coworker, by going to her session to hear her present a paper for which she is listed as the sole author. Laura's paper is on the use of relaxation techniques to decrease muscle tone. You are shocked to discover that Laura's presentation sounds almost identical to an inservice given by a fieldwork student almost 6 months ago.*

See Pages 93-110 for Ethical Dilemma Worksheets

Dilemma 32: *You were Mrs. Anderson's treating therapist in Really Really Rehabilitation Hospital. Several weeks after her discharge Mrs. Anderson comes in to see you. She was shocked by the amount of her bill for therapy services. You are a relatively new therapist. You call your supervisor who quickly tells you to explain to Mrs. Anderson that she should not be concerned about the bill because Medicare will pay the entire bill. The bill is very high and before this, you never knew exactly how much therapy services cost. You relay to Mrs. Anderson your supervisor's explanation. Mrs. Anderson replies that she does not care who pays the bill, she still feels it is not reasonable and not accurate.*

Dilemma 33: *Mr. Soper comes to the therapy clinic to complain about his bill. You were his treating therapist. Mr. Soper insists he was billed too much for services he said he never received. You review Mr. Soper's bill and compare it with your billing sheets and discover that he is right. There are many more units billed for therapy than you performed. You know you recorded the proper amounts when you submitted your billing.*

Dilemma 34: *You are the director of therapy in a rehabilitation hospital. Mr. Miller, a former patient, comes to you to complain about his therapy bill. You review his bill, the billing sheets, and the chart and discover that all of the therapeutic recreation services were billed to your discipline because Medicare, Medicaid, and private insurance do not pay for the services provided by therapeutic recreation.*

Dilemma 35: *You just got a wonderful new job that pays extremely well—more than most of your friends are paid. This is your first job since graduating. You have relocated your family to take the job. After 2 weeks of orientation you are assigned to a nursing home as the sole therapist with two aides to assist you. The caseload is very large. The only way all of the patients can be seen at the frequency ordered by the physicians is to have each aide treat the same number of patients per day as you. You do not think you can properly supervise the aides under these circumstances.*

Dilemma 36: *Mrs. Booker comes to the outpatient department of the hospital where you work. You discover Mrs. Booker's insurance covers outpatient therapy for another discipline but not therapy provided by your discipline. You inform the director. She tells you not to worry because if you treat the patient, the hospital will bill it as the other therapy anyway so the treatment will be paid.*

Dilemma 37: *A medical equipment company offers you a great deal. For every piece of equipment you order for your patients, the company will give you points toward a trip to Hawaii. You have always wanted to go to Hawaii.*

See Pages 93-110 for Ethical Dilemma Worksheets

Dilemma 38: *Your colleague, Mike, is a member of a white supremacist group. From time to time, he has offered you white supremacist literature to read. Mrs. Washington, a 52-year-old African American woman, is referred to therapy. The supervisor assigns Mrs. Washington to Mike. You notice that Mike is often rude to Mrs. Washington. You have also noticed that his treatment is not always appropriate to Mrs. Washington's diagnosis.*

Dilemma 39: *You work in a pediatric setting. You are working with a child in the same area where Karen is treating a child who is severely developmentally disabled. Karen is new to the facility. You are watching her out of the corner of your eye as she works with the child. You notice she is acting inappropriately with the child. She is trying to get the child to keep his head up by flicking the child in the face with her thumb and forefinger. She also appears to be hitting the child. Finally, she picks up the child and shakes him. You see his neck jerk back and he begins to have a seizure. Karen calls for help for the seizure. You later read the incident report and there is no mention of the shaking and other abusive behavior.*

Dilemma 40: *You work in an industrial medicine clinic. One of your clients/patients, Al, wants to return to work. He works hard in your program and you know from your experience he is honest, hard-working, and motivated. However, the workers' compensation carrier will not authorize the diagnostic tests Al needs. His employer will not make the reasonable accommodations you have recommended to enable him to return to work. You know from experience his problems with the carrier and the employer would best be solved if he had a lawyer. He keeps asking you what he can do to get out of his predicament. Although you know a lawyer will improve the situation and ultimately get Al back to work, you are not sure whether you should tell him to get a lawyer. The workers' compensation carrier is paying for the services you are providing to Al and also provides insurance coverage to your employer. You are not sure who your client really is in this situation.*

Dilemma 41: *For 6 weeks you have been working with a young girl, Sarah, who had surgery 4 months ago for a brain tumor. She has made a remarkable recovery. She is walking and her cognitive and perceptual abilities are intact. Her right hand has increased tone and is held in a fisted position with the wrist flexed. The previous therapist was working with Sarah on changing hand dominance, which, in the process, further increased the tone. Although Sarah's hand is nonfunctional at this point, she does have some active finger extension. You believe Sarah needs a splint to decrease the muscle tone and maintain the integrity of the wrist. You call Sarah's neurologist, introduce yourself, and request orders for the splint. He raises his voice and asks you who you think you are, demanding a prescription from him for a splint. He tells you the patient does not need the splint and hangs up the telephone. You know that Sarah will benefit greatly from the splint, which will be the first step in making her right hand functional.*

Dilemma 42: *Susie is a nurse in the outpatient center where you work and a very good friend of Mark, another therapist in your department. Susie was in a car accident 3 weeks ago. She comes into the department to visit Mark during a break complaining about her sore neck. You look over toward Mark and Susie and notice Mark doing soft tissue mobilization on Susie's neck. Your state licensure law requires a physician's prescription or referral before initiating this type of treatment. You know that Mark does not have a physician's referral to provide this treatment to Susie.*

See Pages 93-110 for Ethical Dilemma Worksheets

Dilemma 43: *You work in a long-term care facility that has a restorative therapy program. Lately you have been getting pressure to put a minimum of 40 patients per month in the restorative therapy program. The nursing home administrator tells you the nursing home "accidentally" billed the intermediary for 40 patients, even though only 38 patients were on the program. The administrator wants you to help convince a therapist to write backdated notes for the two patients who were not on the program but were "accidentally" billed for the service. He assures you no one will be harmed by this. You have the feeling that your job and the other therapist's job are on the line if you do not comply with the administrator's request.*

Dilemma 44: *You work in a long-term care facility that has a restorative therapy program. Lately you have been getting pressure to put a minimum of 40 patients per month in the restorative therapy program. You cannot identify 40 residents who meet the criteria of having significant potential for this program. You have the feeling that your job and the other therapist's job are on the line if you do not meet this monthly quota.*

Dilemma 45: *You are working in a subacute rehabilitation unit as a staff therapist. You notice that one of the more experienced therapists always calls for a nurse when one of her patients needs to go to the bathroom. You have seen her leave patients to sit and wait for the nurse for more than 15 minutes. You have seen patients soil themselves while waiting and miss their therapy sessions while nursing cleaned them up. What bothers you the most is that this therapist never works with the patients on transfers to the toilet or any activities of daily living related to hygiene, such as toileting and bathing.*

Dilemma 46: *You work in a rehabilitation center and are treating a patient recovering from a stroke who is covered by an HMO. The patient has had five treatment sessions. During those sessions, the patient made excellent progress. She plans to return home to live with her husband. She continues to have problems with sitting balance, transfers, and hygiene activities and requires further treatment. You call the patient's primary care physician to authorize more treatment sessions and the physician refuses to authorize the additional treatment. The patient will not make further progress without this treatment.*

Dilemma 47: *You work in a children's hospital and share a caseload with a part-time therapist. The part-time therapist is chronically behind on paperwork. She does not write up her evaluations for several days and you are expected to treat these children with no evaluation information about them. You have spoken to this therapist about the lack of documentation. She tells you that seeing the patient is more important than doing the paperwork and she does not have time to do both. You have tried to discuss the issue with your supervisor, but she does not see this as a problem. You are concerned about treating these children without having any information about them.*

See Pages 93-110 for Ethical Dilemma Worksheets

Dilemma 48: *You receive a referral for a patient recovering from hand surgery for a flexor tendon repair. The patient is insured through a managed care plan. The referral requests that the therapist fabricate a custom splint for the flexor tendon repair but does not request any therapy. You call the case manager at the managed care organization who tells you the company will not authorize any therapy—just the splint. You know this patient needs therapy in conjunction with the splint.*

Dilemma 49: *You have provided therapy for Mary's torn rotator cuff. So far, you have treated her for six visits, the amount authorized by her primary care physician. You call the physician for authorization to get more therapy visits for Mary, knowing the published plan cap is 15 visits per year. The physician refuses to authorize more visits. He tells you to write a discharge summary and document that the patient no longer needs treatment. However, you know the patient needs more therapy.*

Dilemma 50: *Your department has a new policy. You may treat patients who are not insured by an HMO for up to 2 hours per day, which is no change from the previous policy. However, HMO patients may only be seen for a maximum of two units per day. One unit equals a 15-minute treatment. Sue, an HMO patient, is a 32-year-old mother of two with a traumatic brain injury from a recent car accident. She has great potential for improvement and good endurance. You know she really needs 2 hours per day of treatment.*

Dilemma 51: *While you are providing passive motion to a patient with flexor tendon lacerations, the patient reveals to you that he injured himself when he broke a window while attempting to break into a house. You joke that he should have remembered his keys, and he goes on to say, "It wasn't my house." You tell him you need to focus on the therapy. When the patient leaves, you are concerned you should do something with the information he disclosed.*

Dilemma 52: *You are working with a patient, Sarah, who has suffered from depression on and off over the last several years. She comes in for treatment one day appearing very down. Sarah relates to you several very stressful events in her life that she finds herself struggling to face at present. She tells you she is ready to give up. She asks you, "Everything I tell you is confidential, right?" You reply affirmatively, assuring Sarah that everything she tells you is confidential. Sarah then tells you that she plans to kill herself if things do not get better for her soon. She cannot take it anymore. She has carefully thought out how she will kill herself and she tells you that this thought is bringing her peace.*

Dilemma 53: *You receive a referral from a family practice doctor for therapy for a patient diagnosed with carpal tunnel syndrome. The referral states, "Make carpal tunnel splint and educate patient." However, based on the history and your assessment, you are pretty sure the patient has a trigger finger and not carpal tunnel.*

See Pages 93-110 for Ethical Dilemma Worksheets

Dilemma 54: *You have treated Ashley's traumatic hand injury for 2 months now and anticipate at least another 2 months of treatment. You find Ashley attractive, and while performing Ashley's hand therapy you have fantasized about a future together. The opportunity finally arises for the two of you to go out to dinner and a movie over the weekend. You have a wonderful time and end up at Ashley's house for a late night snack. One thing leads to another and you find yourself faced with an invitation to spend the night, but not on the couch. Your fantasies seem to be coming true.*

Dilemma 55: *Your facility wants to make sure it can show progress in all patients it treats. To document progress for Medicare patients, the department adopts an unwritten policy of recording a 1/2 lower muscle grade for manual muscle testing on all initial evaluations.*

Dilemma 56: *You begin to work at a long-term care facility. You are the only licensed therapist in the facility. There are no licensed assistants working in the facility, but there are several aides. At the end of the first week, the aides come to you with their typed notes for your signature. You were not even present when these aides performed their "treatment."*

Dilemma 57: *You do some fill-in work in a clinic. The clinic is very busy. You finally get a short break and you inquire about documentation requirements. They tell you not to worry, "We will do your notes for you."*

Dilemma 58: *You witness a therapist teaching a level one fieldwork student to use ultrasound to carry out a treatment on one of the assigned patients. You know the student has not had any formal training in the use of electric modalities.*

Dilemma 59: *You are assigned a patient who had been treated by another therapist. You discover the splint made by the previous therapist was harming the patient and the patient has a large ulcerated sore on the dorsum of her hand under the splint.*

Dilemma 60: *You are a recent graduate. Your facility expects you to see three patients at one time. For a number of reasons, you do not feel comfortable seeing three patients at the same time. You worry about spending enough time with each patient, about the quality of care you can provide under the circumstances, and about potential billing problems.*

See Pages 93-110 for Ethical Dilemma Worksheets

Dilemma 61: *You work in a hospital rehabilitation department. The employee health department asks you to assist in the employee selection process. Employee health wants you to set up a program to screen out all nurses and nurse's aides who have a history of back injuries or workers' compensation claims.*

Dilemma 62: *Mr. Robinson comes to outpatient services for therapy. During your initial evaluation, you ask Mr. Robinson if he previously received your type of therapy. His reply of "sort of" makes you curious. After further inquiry, Mr. Robinson informs you that he had a home health therapist. At the end of each visit, the home health therapist gave Mr. Robinson two treatment verification slips to sign—one for this type of therapy and one for another type of therapy. You know the home health therapist who treated Mr. Robinson and also know the therapist is not licensed—let alone trained—in both disciplines.*

Dilemma 63: *Your facility needs a supervisor in the neurology section of the therapy department. You have never worked in neurology and know little about it. The director of rehabilitation offers you the position. The position comes with a substantial raise.*

Dilemma 64: *You have worked in the same facility for about 3 years. All of a sudden you realize that male therapists with less experience have consistently been promoted over female therapists with more experience.*

Dilemma 65: *You are the supervisor in a rather large therapy department. You are recruiting for several additional positions. The "higher ups" tell you that when you interview male therapists, you should offer them at least $5,000 more in salary than you offer the female applicants.*

Dilemma 66: *You are treating a home health patient. At the end of the session, as you ready yourself to leave, the patient's wife asks you if she can have a ride to the grocery store, which she knows is on your way to your next patient.*

Dilemma 67: *You are treating a home health patient in the patient's home. The patient is post-CVA and takes many medications, some by hyperalimentation, a machine that needs electricity for operation. Just as the session is about to end, the power goes out in one of the area's summer "brown-outs." Nobody else is home with the patient except you.*

See Pages 93-110 for Ethical Dilemma Worksheets

Dilemma 68: *Your employer tells you that you are to bill all evaluations for 12 units regardless of the time spent with the patient. However, you complete most of your initial evaluations in 8 units. You keep receiving memoranda reminding you that you are not keeping up with expected production.*

Dilemma 69: *You observe a therapist performing a routine procedure on a patient incorrectly. In fact, the patient is complaining that the procedure is hurting him. You are concerned that if the therapist continues to treat the patient in the same manner, the patient will very likely suffer an injury.*

Dilemma 70: *Dr. Zaborowzki referred Mr. Smith to you for a specific treatment modality. In your review of Mr. Smith's chart you discover Mr. Smith's diagnosis. You are aware that the specific treatment ordered by Dr. Zaborowzki is contraindicated for persons with Mr. Smith's diagnosis.*

Dilemma 71: *You work in an inpatient facility. One of your coworkers does home health part-time in addition to being employed full-time at your facility. You have periodically observed this therapist completing her home health progress notes while on duty at the facility.*

Dilemma 72: *You work for an innovative private therapy company that will pay you $2.00 for every treatment unit over 100 units that you bill each week. The company will pay you an additional $4.00 for each unit over 120 units that you bill each week.*

Dilemma 73: *You work for an innovative therapy company that will pay you $2.00 for every treatment unit over 100 units that you bill each week. The company will also pay you $4.00 for each unit over 120 units that you bill each week. Your coworker inflates her units by billing for units that she did not provide.*

Dilemma 74: *During one of your clinical affiliations (internships), you notice that your supervisor regularly documents patient treatment units and progress before treating the patient.*

Dilemma 75: *You are a staff therapist. You notice that your immediate supervisor regularly bills patients for more treatment units than were provided by you and others.*

See Pages 93-110 for Ethical Dilemma Worksheets

Dilemma 76: *During your clinical affiliation (internship), Mrs. Higginbotham asks you how much experience you have had with the particular treatment you are providing to her.*

Dilemma 77: *Mr. Marcus is 75 years old. He regularly attends outpatient therapy. On each of his last three visits you have observed that Mr. Marcus had large bruises on his back, arms, and legs. You think that some of the marks resemble handprints. You know that Mr. Marcus lives alone and that a home health aide visits him daily.*

Dilemma 78: *You notice that 5-year-old Bobby has repeatedly showed up for outpatient therapy with bruises on his arms, legs, and back. Today he showed up with a 2-inch cut on his forehead and bruises on his face. You suspect that the injuries are a result of physical abuse. The facility administration refuses to allow you to report your suspicion.*

Dilemma 79: *It is summer and your coworkers have been taking their family vacations. Your supervisor arranged to have therapists from XYZ agency cover the caseloads of your vacationing coworkers. Every day the agency sends a different therapist to your facility. In addition, the therapists sent by the agency were trained in a foreign country. You do not believe the therapists are qualified to work with the patients.*

Dilemma 80: *You were recently hired to work at Dynamic & Wonderful Healthcare Facility. You are eager to make a positive impression on your coworkers and supervisor. To facilitate the cumbersome evaluation process used by the Dynamic staff, you offer a copy of an evaluation form you developed when you worked for Therapeutic Excellence. The evaluation form has a copyright symbol (©) located on the bottom of each page beside Therapeutic Excellence's name.*

Dilemma 81: *Mr. Dean has a driver's license but has severe perceptual deficits as a result of head trauma. You know Mr. Dean cannot drive safely, but you are concerned that if you take Mr. Dean's license away, it will severely impair his ability to work, shop, and manage his daily life.*

Dilemma 82: *Mrs. Stansa had a CVA. She did not renew her driver's license after she had her stroke. Today she arrives for therapy and proudly announces, "I drove my daughter's brand new car to therapy today!"*

See Pages 93-110 for Ethical Dilemma Worksheets

Dilemma 83: *A patient is in her bed with no clothes on and is fully exposed to passersby. Her call light is on but staff is not responding. You know the light has been on for 20 minutes. You are at the nurses' station. The buzzer to the patient's room is still beeping.*

Dilemma 84: *You observed a 20-minute therapy session with a child. After the 20-minute session, the child's therapist asks the teacher to sign a verification stating that the child participated in 30 minutes of therapy.*

Dilemma 85: *A therapist coworker calls the office and notifies you she is going to be late. She asks you to please start seeing her patients for her and you agree to do so. The therapist arrives to work 3 hours later.*

Dilemma 86: *Over the last 4 days, every time you have seen Mr. Blumberg he has been restrained while sitting in his wheelchair. You know no one has ever performed a restraint evaluation on Mr. Blumberg.*

Dilemma 87: *The supervising therapist always documents that he has provided 30-minute treatment sessions to every patient. You know that the supervisor frequently sees patients for less than 30 minutes. He also sometimes sees patients for more than 30 minutes.*

Dilemma 88: *Mrs. Vasquez calls you to complain about the number of hours she was billed for your therapy. When you review your billing records, you discover that she has been charged many more hours than what your records indicate. This is the fourth complaint of this kind that you have received, and the fourth time that the patient's actual bill has seriously exceeded the number of treatment units you had recorded.*

Dilemma 89: *A certified/licensed therapist is on vacation. To avoid scheduling problems and to ensure that all patients continue to receive services, an aide has been assigned to cover the vacationing therapist's caseload.*

Dilemma 90: *A child's individual educational plan (IEP) indicates that he is to receive individual treatment. The child is always treated in group sessions because it is more time and cost effective. The child is always billed for individual therapy.*

See Pages 93-110 for Ethical Dilemma Worksheets

Dilemma 91: *Several therapists are collaborating in running a cooking group to facilitate multiple therapeutic goals (ambulation, speech, fine motor skills, cognition). Therapist Whitehall refers a new patient to the cooking group. Therapist Nitkin pulls therapist Whitehall aside and states, "Your patient cannot be in this cooking group because she has AIDS."*

Dilemma 92: *Several therapists are collaborating in running a cooking group to facilitate multiple therapeutic goals (ambulation, speech, fine motor skills, cognition). Therapist Whitehall refers a new patient to the cooking group. In front of another patient, therapist Littlesunday blurts out, "That person has AIDS! He has AIDS!"*

Dilemma 93: *Patients and family members are sitting at a table in the treatment area. At the same table, a therapist is writing progress notes in several patient charts. The therapist walks away, leaving the patient charts on the table. Fifteen minutes have passed and the therapist has not returned.*

Dilemma 94: *Under the prospective payment system in long-term care, the results of a patient's therapy evaluations, including the number of minutes each therapy service treats the patient, are put on the minimum data set (MDS) form. You discover that in your facility, the results of the MDS consistently indicate the patient is functioning at a significantly lower level than your evaluation indicates. Further, the MDS form also indicates a higher number of minutes of treatment time for your therapy service than your evaluation results warrant.*

Dilemma 95: *You apply for a position you found advertised in a national publication. Two weeks after mailing your application you receive a letter from the prospective employer stating, "We tried to contact you on January 3, January 14, and January 28, and were unable to reach you. Therefore we assume you are no longer interested in the position opening and have removed your name from our applicant pool." You never received a message and your caller ID never indicated a call was received from this employer. You call the employer to indicate your continued interest. A clerk informs you that the position is not really available and that the ad was placed to comply with state and federal regulations. The employer already hired a foreign therapist and is awaiting immigration approval.*

Dilemma 96: *Your employer wants you to sign progress notes written by a newly graduated therapist who has not yet passed the board examination. You have worked with this therapist and, in your opinion, the therapist is a competent entry-level practitioner.*

See Pages 93-110 for Ethical Dilemma Worksheets

Dilemma 97: *Your employer wants you to sign progress notes written by a newly graduated therapist who has not yet passed the board examination. You work in the same room with the therapist and have observed all treatment sessions.*

Dilemma 98: *Your employer wants you to sign progress notes written by a newly graduated therapist who has not yet passed the board examination. You have not seen the therapist work with patients.*

Dilemma 99: *Your supervisor wants you to cosign progress notes written by a certified, licensed, or registered assistant. The assistant provides therapy to patients in the facility 5 days per week. You are only in the facility 3 days per week.*

Dilemma 100: *Your facility has hired a full-time certified/licensed assistant to provide patient treatment in one of its programs. A contract therapist completes all patient evaluations for the program and comes in one time per month to cosign the assistant's notes. Other than the evaluation, the therapist does not see the patients. You are a therapist who provides services in another program in the facility.*

Dilemma 101: *A therapist coworker is going on vacation. The therapist arranged for another therapist to come in and sign the certified/licensed assistant's notes. This other therapist did not evaluate and has never seen the patients.*

Dilemma 102: *You have replaced a therapist who moved out of town. On Monday, you tell Ms. Merriweather you will be back to see her on Wednesday and Friday. Ms. Merriweather tells you that her former therapist only saw her two times a week, on Mondays and Wednesdays. Ms. Merriweather's prescription requires therapy three times per week.*

Dilemma 103: *You answer the telephone in the clinic. The caller asks to speak to the clinical fieldwork supervisor. The supervisor takes the call and you overhear her state, "Yes, Mary was a student here. She had some difficulties, but she has a learning disability and if you work with her she'll work out for you."*

See Pages 93-110 for Ethical Dilemma Worksheets

Dilemma 104: *In acute rehabilitation facilities, a patient must have 3 hours of therapy per day to stay in the facility. Paul has orders for two therapy services twice a day. However, Paul consistently refuses to participate in one of the two therapies. Your supervisor has asked you to document the time you spend trying to persuade him to come to therapy as "cognitive training."*

Dilemma 105: *Abraham has been employed at your facility for 6 months and is well respected by both the patients and staff. At lunch, Samantha leans over to you and says, "Too bad about that guy Abraham. I'd go out with him except that he is manic depressive and is wild when he doesn't take his medication."*

Dilemma 106: *A therapist worked for a rehabilitation company in Wisconsin. The therapist moved from Wisconsin to your facility in Utah and took with her the restorative therapy program manual from the previous employer. The previous employer was well known for providing training programs around the country using the techniques in its restorative therapy program. The therapist has approached you to implement the program in your facility. You attended one of the workshops and know that the information belongs to the therapist's previous employer.*

Dilemma 107: *You work in a rehabilitation center attached to a large hospital. Currently, the rehabilitation employees' identification badges include their name, credentials, position, and title. The rehabilitation director announces a new policy: Starting next week, all employees who work in the rehabilitation center will wear identification badges that include only their name and the designation "rehab."*

Dilemma 108: *You receive a subpoena from an attorney who wants to take your deposition. The case concerns a child who was injured in an accident some 4 years ago. You evaluated the child once almost 3 1/2 years ago. Although you performed an evaluation, you never treated the child and you do not remember anything about the child.*

Dilemma 109: *You are an academic fieldwork coordinator at a university. One of your students who will be beginning her fieldwork/internship tells you she will not inform her clinical supervisor of her learning disability. This student got through the classroom portion of her education with the assistance of numerous reasonable accommodations. Without these reasonable accommodations, the student will not have the advantages she had in the classroom.*

See Pages 93-110 for Ethical Dilemma Worksheets

Dilemma 110: *You are an academic fieldwork coordinator at a university. One of your students, who has a learning disability, finds herself failing her fieldwork/internship. Three weeks after the student begins her fieldwork, you receive a telephone call from the clinical supervisor at the fieldwork site informing you that the student is failing. She makes no mention of the student's learning disability.*

Dilemma 111: *You are a clinical fieldwork coordinator at a major hospital. One of the students simply cannot perform up to par. Based on her performance, including, among other things, numerous spelling errors in documentation, you suspect the student has a learning disability. The student has never shared this with you, but you are very certain of your "diagnosis."*

Dilemma 112: *You work in a very large rehabilitation department. As head of the department, you hire a new therapist. She has worked as a therapist for 10 years. After hiring the therapist, you discover she has a condition that does not allow her to perform any patient transfers.*

Dilemma 113: *You work in the public school system. You have treated Billy for 2 years. He has reached a plateau and you feel he can no longer benefit from therapy. After you discharge Billy from therapy, the principal comes to you and screams to put the child back in therapy because Billy's father, a very important person in the community, wants Billy to have more therapy.*

Dilemma 114: *You work in the public school system. You are overwhelmed with students to treat because there are not enough staff. You are told by your supervisor to see the patients in groups. Several of the children need one-on-one treatment in order to benefit from therapy.*

Dilemma 115: *Mr. Murphy is a new patient. During your first visit with him, you strongly suspect Mr. Murphy is having psychotic episodes or periods of dementia. You believe he is not competent to give informed consent. On investigation, you discover he has never been declared incompetent. Therefore, he does not have a guardian.*

See Pages 93-110 for Ethical Dilemma Worksheets

Section

III

Ethical Dilemma Worksheets

◆ Ethical Dilemma Worksheet ◆

1. **What is the problem?**

   _____

2. **What are the facts of the situation?**

   _____

3. **Who are the interested parties?**

   Facility?
   _____

   Patient?
   _____

   Other therapists?
   _____

   Observers?
   _____

   Payers?
   _____

   Others:
   _____

4. **What is the nature of their interest? Why is this a problem?**

   Professional
   _____

   Personal
   _____

   Business
   _____

   Economic
   _____

   Intellectual
   _____

   Societal

Interested Parties	Their Interests

5. **Ethical?**

   Does it violate a professional code of ethics? Which section(s)?
   _____

   Does it violate moral, social, or religious values?

6. **Is there a legal issue?**

_____

Practice Act/Licensure law and regulations? Section(s)?

_____

Check the CELIBATE checklist for other possible legal issues:

_____

7. **Do I need more information?**

_____

What information do I need?

_____

Is there a treatment, policy, procedure, law, regulation, or document that I do not know about?

_____

Can I obtain a copy of the treatment, policy, procedure, law, regulation, or document in writing?

_____

Do I need to research the issue further?

_____

Do I need to consult with a mentor, an expert in this area, and/or a lawyer?

_____

8. **Brainstorm possible action steps**

_____

9. **Analyze action steps**

_____

Eliminate the obvious wrong choices

_____

How will each alternative affect my patients, other interested parties, and me?

_____

Do your choices abide by the code of ethics?

_____

Do your choices abide by the practice act and regulations?

_____

Are my choices consistent with my moral, religious, and social beliefs?

_____

Eliminate obviously wrong or impossible choices

_____

10. **Choose your course of action**

_____

The Rotary four-way test:

_____

Is it the _truth_?

_____

Is is _fair_ to all concerned?

_____

Will it build _goodwill_ and _better friendship_?

_____

Will it be _beneficial_ to all concerned?

_____

Is it win-win?

_____

How do you feel about your course of action?

_____

◆ Ethical Dilemma Worksheet ◆

1. What is the problem?

_____

2. What are the facts of the situation?

_____

3. Who are the interested parties?

Facility?
_____

Patient?
_____

Other therapists?
_____

Observers?
_____

Payers?
_____

Others:
_____

4. What is the nature of their interest? Why is this a problem?

Professional
_____

Personal
_____

Business
_____

Economic
_____

Intellectual
_____

Societal

Interested Parties	Their Interests

5. Ethical?

Does it violate a professional code of ethics? Which section(s)?
_____

Does it violate moral, social, or religious values?

6. Is there a legal issue?

Practice Act/Licensure law and regulations? Section(s)?

Check the CELIBATE checklist for other possible legal issues:

7. Do I need more information?

What information do I need?

Is there a treatment, policy, procedure, law, regulation, or document that I do not know about?

Can I obtain a copy of the treatment, policy, procedure, law, regulation, or document in writing?

Do I need to research the issue further?

Do I need to consult with a mentor, an expert in this area, and/or a lawyer?

8. Brainstorm possible action steps

9. Analyze action steps

Eliminate the obvious wrong choices

How will each alternative affect my patients, other interested parties, and me?

Do your choices abide by the code of ethics?

Do your choices abide by the practice act and regulations?

Are my choices consistent with my moral, religious, and social beliefs?

Eliminate obviously wrong or impossible choices

10. Choose your course of action

The Rotary four-way test:

Is it the *truth*?

Is is *fair* to all concerned?

Will it build *goodwill* and *better friendship*?

Will it be *beneficial* to all concerned?

Is it win-win?

How do you feel about your course of action?

◆ Ethical Dilemma Worksheet ◆

1. **What is the problem?**

   _____

2. **What are the facts of the situation?**

   _____

3. **Who are the interested parties?**

   _____

   Facility?

   _____

   Patient?

   _____

   Other therapists?

   _____

   Observers?

   _____

   Payers?

   _____

   Others:

   _____

4. **What is the nature of their interest? Why is this a problem?**

   _____

   Professional

   _____

   Personal

   _____

   Business

   _____

   Economic

   _____

   Intellectual

   _____

   Societal

Interested Parties	Their Interests

5. **Ethical?**

   _____

   Does it violate a professional code of ethics? Which section(s)?

   _____

   Does it violate moral, social, or religious values?

6. **Is there a legal issue?**

Practice Act/Licensure law and regulations? Section(s)?

Check the CELIBATE checklist for other possible legal issues:

7. **Do I need more information?**

What information do I need?

Is there a treatment, policy, procedure, law, regulation, or document that I do not know about?

Can I obtain a copy of the treatment, policy, procedure, law, regulation, or document in writing?

Do I need to research the issue further?

Do I need to consult with a mentor, an expert in this area, and/or a lawyer?

8. **Brainstorm possible action steps**

9. **Analyze action steps**

Eliminate the obvious wrong choices

How will each alternative affect my patients, other interested parties, and me?

Do your choices abide by the code of ethics?

Do your choices abide by the practice act and regulations?

Are my choices consistent with my moral, religious, and social beliefs?

Eliminate obviously wrong or impossible choices

10. **Choose your course of action**

The Rotary four-way test:

Is it the *truth*?

Is is *fair* to all concerned?

Will it build *goodwill* and *better friendship*?

Will it be *beneficial* to all concerned?

Is it win-win?

How do you feel about your course of action?

◆ Ethical Dilemma Worksheet ◆

1. **What is the problem?**

_____

2. **What are the facts of the situation?**

_____

3. **Who are the interested parties?**

_____

Facility?

_____

Patient?

_____

Other therapists?

_____

Observers?

_____

Payers?

_____

Others:

_____

4. **What is the nature of their interest? Why is this a problem?**

_____

Professional

_____

Personal

_____

Business

_____

Economic

_____

Intellectual

_____

Societal

Interested Parties	Their Interests

5. **Ethical?**

_____

Does it violate a professional code of ethics? Which section(s)?

_____

Does it violate moral, social, or religious values?

6. **Is there a legal issue?**

Practice Act/Licensure law and regulations? Section(s)?

Check the CELIBATE checklist for other possible legal issues:

7. **Do I need more information?**

What information do I need?

Is there a treatment, policy, procedure, law, regulation, or document that I do not know about?

Can I obtain a copy of the treatment, policy, procedure, law, regulation, or document in writing?

Do I need to research the issue further?

Do I need to consult with a mentor, an expert in this area, and/or a lawyer?

8. **Brainstorm possible action steps**

9. **Analyze action steps**

Eliminate the obvious wrong choices

How will each alternative affect my patients, other interested parties, and me?

Do your choices abide by the code of ethics?

Do your choices abide by the practice act and regulations?

Are my choices consistent with my moral, religious, and social beliefs?

Eliminate obviously wrong or impossible choices

10. **Choose your course of action**

The Rotary four-way test:

Is it the *truth*?

Is is *fair* to all concerned?

Will it build *goodwill* and *better friendship*?

Will it be *beneficial* to all concerned?

Is it win-win?

How do you feel about your course of action?

◆ Ethical Dilemma Worksheet ◆

1. **What is the problem?**

   _____

2. **What are the facts of the situation?**

   _____

3. **Who are the interested parties?**

   Facility?
   _____

   Patient?
   _____

   Other therapists?
   _____

   Observers?
   _____

   Payers?
   _____

   Others:
   _____

4. **What is the nature of their interest? Why is this a problem?**

   Professional
   _____

   Personal
   _____

   Business
   _____

   Economic
   _____

   Intellectual
   _____

   Societal

Interested Parties	Their Interests

5. **Ethical?**

   Does it violate a professional code of ethics? Which section(s)?
   _____

   Does it violate moral, social, or religious values?
   _____

6. Is there a legal issue?

Practice Act/Licensure law and regulations? Section(s)?

Check the CELIBATE checklist for other possible legal issues:

7. Do I need more information?

What information do I need?

Is there a treatment, policy, procedure, law, regulation, or document that I do not know about?

Can I obtain a copy of the treatment, policy, procedure, law, regulation, or document in writing?

Do I need to research the issue further?

Do I need to consult with a mentor, an expert in this area, and/or a lawyer?

8. Brainstorm possible action steps

9. Analyze action steps

Eliminate the obvious wrong choices

How will each alternative affect my patients, other interested parties, and me?

Do your choices abide by the code of ethics?

Do your choices abide by the practice act and regulations?

Are my choices consistent with my moral, religious, and social beliefs?

Eliminate obviously wrong or impossible choices

10. Choose your course of action

The Rotary four-way test:

Is it the *truth*?

Is is *fair* to all concerned?

Will it build *goodwill* and *better friendship*?

Will it be *beneficial* to all concerned?

Is it win-win?

How do you feel about your course of action?

◆ Ethical Dilemma Worksheet ◆

1. **What is the problem?**

_____

2. **What are the facts of the situation?**

_____

3. **Who are the interested parties?**

   Facility?
   _____

   Patient?
   _____

   Other therapists?
   _____

   Observers?
   _____

   Payers?
   _____

   Others:
   _____

4. **What is the nature of their interest? Why is this a problem?**

   Professional
   _____

   Personal
   _____

   Business
   _____

   Economic
   _____

   Intellectual
   _____

   Societal

Interested Parties	Their Interests

5. **Ethical?**

   Does it violate a professional code of ethics? Which section(s)?
   _____

   Does it violate moral, social, or religious values?

6. **Is there a legal issue?**

Practice Act/Licensure law and regulations? Section(s)?

Check the CELIBATE checklist for other possible legal issues:

7. **Do I need more information?**

What information do I need?

Is there a treatment, policy, procedure, law, regulation, or document that I do not know about?

Can I obtain a copy of the treatment, policy, procedure, law, regulation, or document in writing?

Do I need to research the issue further?

Do I need to consult with a mentor, an expert in this area, and/or a lawyer?

8. **Brainstorm possible action steps**

9. **Analyze action steps**

Eliminate the obvious wrong choices

How will each alternative affect my patients, other interested parties, and me?

Do your choices abide by the code of ethics?

Do your choices abide by the practice act and regulations?

Are my choices consistent with my moral, religious, and social beliefs?

Eliminate obviously wrong or impossible choices

10. **Choose your course of action**

The Rotary four-way test:

Is it the *truth*?

Is is *fair* to all concerned?

Will it build *goodwill* and *better friendship*?

Will it be *beneficial* to all concerned?

Is it win-win?

How do you feel about your course of action?

◆ Ethical Dilemma Worksheet ◆

1. What is the problem?

_____

2. What are the facts of the situation?

_____

3. Who are the interested parties?

_____

Facility?

_____

Patient?

_____

Other therapists?

_____

Observers?

_____

Payers?

_____

Others:

_____

4. What is the nature of their interest? Why is this a problem?

_____

Professional

_____

Personal

_____

Business

_____

Economic

_____

Intellectual

_____

Societal

Interested Parties	Their Interests

5. Ethical?

_____

Does it violate a professional code of ethics? Which section(s)?

_____

Does it violate moral, social, or religious values?

6. Is there a legal issue?

Practice Act/Licensure law and regulations? Section(s)?

Check the CELIBATE checklist for other possible legal issues:

7. Do I need more information?

What information do I need?

Is there a treatment, policy, procedure, law, regulation, or document that I do not know about?

Can I obtain a copy of the treatment, policy, procedure, law, regulation, or document in writing?

Do I need to research the issue further?

Do I need to consult with a mentor, an expert in this area, and/or a lawyer?

8. Brainstorm possible action steps

9. Analyze action steps

Eliminate the obvious wrong choices

How will each alternative affect my patients, other interested parties, and me?

Do your choices abide by the code of ethics?

Do your choices abide by the practice act and regulations?

Are my choices consistent with my moral, religious, and social beliefs?

Eliminate obviously wrong or impossible choices

10. Choose your course of action

The Rotary four-way test:

Is it the *truth*?

Is is *fair* to all concerned?

Will it build *goodwill* and *better friendship*?

Will it be *beneficial* to all concerned?

Is it win-win?

How do you feel about your course of action?

SECTION
IV
Appendices

A

AOTA, APTA, and ASHA Codes of Ethics

AOTA CODE OF ETHICS

Please note: A revised Code of Ethics was being voted on at the time of this printing. Once approved, a copy of the new Code of Ethics can be obtained by contacting the AOTA at:

4720 Montgomery Lane
P.O. Box 31220
Bethesda, MD 20824-1220.
301-652-2682
1-800-377-8555
www.aota.org

The American Occupational Therapy Association's Code of Ethics is a public statement of the values and principles used in promoting and maintaining high standards of behavior in occupational therapy. The American Occupational Therapy Association and its members are committed to furthering people's ability to function within their total environment. To this end, occupational therapy personnel provide services for individuals in any stage of health and illness, to institutions, to other professionals and colleagues, to students, and to the general public.

The Occupational Therapy Code of Ethics, is a set of principles that applies to occupational therapy personnel at all levels. The roles of practitioner (reg-istered occupational therapist and certified occupational therapy assistant), educator, fieldwork educator, supervisor, administrator, consultant, fieldwork coordinator, faculty program director, researcher/scholar, entrepreneur, student, support staff, and occupational therapy aide are assumed.

Any action that is in violation of the spirit and purpose of this Code shall be considered unethical. To ensure compliance with the Code, enforcement procedures are established and maintained by the Commission on Standards and Ethics. Acceptance of membership in the American Occupational Therapy Association commits members to adherence to the Code of Ethics and its enforcement procedures.

Principle 1. Occupational therapy personnel shall demonstrate a concern for the well- being of the recipients of their services. (beneficence)

A. Occupational therapy personnel shall provide services in an equitable manner for all individuals.

B. Occupational therapy personnel shall maintain relationships that do not exploit the recipient of services sexually, physically, emotionally, financially, socially or in any other manner. Occupational therapy personnel shall avoid those relationships or activities that interfere with professional judgment and objectivity.

C. Occupational therapy personnel shall take all reasonable precautions to avoid harm to the recipient of services or to his or her property.

D. Occupational therapy personnel shall strive to ensure that fees are fair, reasonable, and commensurate with the service performed and are set with due regard for the service recipient's ability to pay.

Principle 2. Occupational therapy personnel shall respect the rights of the recipients of their services. (e.g., autonomy, privacy, confidentiality)

A. Occupational therapy personnel shall collaborate with service recipients or their surrogate(s) in determining goals and priorities throughout the intervention process.

B. Occupational therapy personnel shall fully inform the service recipients of the nature, risks, and potential outcomes of any interventions.

C. Occupational therapy personnel shall obtain informed consent from subjects involved in research activities indicating they have been fully advised of the potential risks and outcomes.

D. Occupational therapy personnel shall respect the individual's right to refuse professional services or involvement in research or educational activities.

E. Occupational therapy personnel shall protect the confidential nature of information gained from educational, practice, research, and investigational activities.

Principle 3. Occupational therapy personnel shall achieve and continually maintain high standards of competence. (duties)

A. Occupational therapy practitioners shall hold the appropriate national and state credentials for providing services.

B. Occupational therapy personnel shall use procedures that conform to the Standards of Practice of the American Occupational Therapy Association.

C. Occupational therapy personnel shall take responsibility for maintaining competence by

participating in professional development and educational activities.

D. Occupational therapy personnel shall perform their duties on the basis of accurate and current information.

E. Occupational therapy practitioners shall protect service recipients by ensuring that duties assumed by or assigned to other occupational therapy personnel are commensurate with their qualifications and experience.

F. Occupational therapy practitioners shall provide appropriate supervision to individuals for whom the practitioners have supervisory responsibility.

G. Occupational therapists shall refer recipients to other service providers or consult with other service providers when additional knowledge and expertise are required.

Principle 4. Occupational therapy personnel shall comply with laws and Association policies guiding the profession of occupational therapy. (justice)

A. Occupational therapy personnel shall understand and abide by applicable Association policies; local, state, and federal laws; and institutional rules.

B. Occupational therapy personnel shall inform employers, employees, and colleagues about those laws and Association policies that apply to the profession of occupational therapy.

C. Occupational therapy practitioners shall require those they supervise in occupational therapy related activities to adhere to the Code of Ethics.

D. Occupational therapy personnel shall accurately record and report all information related to professional activities.

Principle 5. Occupational therapy personnel shall provide accurate information about occupational therapy services. (veracity)

A. Occupational therapy personnel shall accurately represent their qualifications, education, experience, training, and competence.

B. Occupational therapy personnel shall disclose any affiliations that may pose a conflict of interest.

C. Occupational therapy personnel shall refrain from using or participating in the use of any form of communication that contains false, fraudulent, deceptive, or unfair statements or claims.

Principle 6. Occupational therapy personnel shall treat colleagues and other professionals with fairness, discretion, and integrity. (fidelity, veracity)

A. Occupational therapy personnel shall safeguard confidential information about colleagues and staff.

B. Occupational therapy personnel shall accurately represent the qualifications, views, contributions, and findings of colleagues.

C. Occupational therapy personnel shall report any breaches of the Code of Ethics to the appropriate authority.

Author: Commission on Standards and Ethics (SEC); Ruth Hansen, PhD, OT, FAOTA, Chairperson

Approved by the Representative Assembly: 4/77
Revised: 1979, 1988, 1994
Adopted by the Representative Assembly: 7/94

Note: *This document replaces the 1988 Occupational Therapy Code of Ethics, which was rescinded by the 1994 Representative Assembly.*

APTA Code of Ethics

Preamble

This Code of Ethics sets forth ethical principles for the physical therapy profession. Members of this profession are responsible for maintaining and promoting ethical practice. This Code of Ethics, adopted by the American Physical Therapy Association, shall be binding on physical therapists who are members of the Association.

Principle 1

Physical therapists respect the rights and dignity of all individuals.

Principle 2

Physical therapists comply with the laws and regulations governing the practice of physical therapy.

Principle 3

Physical therapists accept responsibility for the exercise of sound judgment.

Principle 4

Physical therapists maintain and promote high standards for physical therapy practice, education, and research.

Principle 5

Physical therapists seek remuneration for their services that is deserved and reasonable.

Principle 6

Physical therapists provide accurate information to the consumer about the profession and about those services they provide.

Principle 7

Physical therapists accept the responsibility to protect the public and the profession from unethical, incompetent, or illegal acts.

Principle 8

Physical therapists participate in efforts to address the health needs of the public.

Reprinted from www.apta.org/Ethics/code_of_ethics.html, with permission of the American Physical Therapy Association.

ASHA Code of Ethics

Preamble

The preservation of the highest standards of integrity and ethical principles is vital to the responsible discharge of obligations in the professions of speech-language pathology and audiology. This Code of Ethics sets forth the fundamental principles and rules considered essential to this purpose.

Every individual who is (a) a member of the American Speech-Language-Hearing Association, whether certified or not, (b) a nonmember holding the Certificate of Clinical Competence from the Association, (c) an applicant for membership or certification, or (d) a Clinical Fellow seeking to fulfill standards for certification shall abide by this Code of Ethics.

Any action that violates the spirit and purpose of this Code shall be considered unethical. Failure to specify any particular responsibility or practice in this Code of Ethics shall not be construed as denial of the existence of such responsibilities or practices.

The fundamentals of ethical conduct are described by Principles of Ethics and by Rules of Ethics as they relate to responsibility to persons served, to the public, and to the professions of speech-language pathology and audiology.

Principles of Ethics, aspirational and inspirational in nature, form the underlying moral basis for the Code of Ethics. Individuals shall observe these principles as affirmative obligations under all conditions of professional activity.

Rules of Ethics are specific statements of minimally acceptable professional conduct or of prohibitions and are applicable to all individuals.

Principle of Ethics I

Individuals shall honor their responsibility to hold paramount the welfare of persons they serve professionally.

Rules of Ethics

A. Individuals shall provide all services competently.

B. Individuals shall use every resource, including referral when appropriate, to ensure that high-quality service is provided.

C. Individuals shall not discriminate in the delivery of professional services on the basis of race or ethnicity, gender, age, religion, national origin, sexual orientation, or disability.

D. Individuals shall fully inform the persons they serve of the nature and possible effects of services rendered and products dispensed.

E. Individuals shall evaluate the effectiveness of services rendered and of products dispensed and shall provide services or dispense products only when benefit can reasonably be expected.

F. Individuals shall not guarantee the results of any treatment or procedure, directly or by implication; however, they may make a reasonable statement of prognosis.

G. Individuals shall not evaluate or treat speech, language, or hearing disorders solely by correspondence.

H. Individuals shall maintain adequate records of professional services rendered and products dispensed and shall allow access to these records when appropriately authorized.

I. Individuals shall not reveal, without authorization, any professional or personal information about the person served professionally, unless required by law to do so, or unless doing so is necessary to protect the welfare of the person or of the community.

J. Individuals shall not charge for services not rendered, nor shall they misrepresent, in any fashion, services rendered or products dispensed.

K. Individuals shall use persons in research or as subjects of teaching demonstrations only with their informed consent.

L. Individuals whose professional services are adversely affected by substance abuse or other health-related conditions shall seek professional assistance and, where appropriate, withdraw from the affected areas of practice.

For purposes of this Code of Ethics, misrepresentation includes any untrue statements or statements that are likely to mislead. Misrepresentation also includes the failure to state any information that is material and that ought, in fairness, to be considered.

Principle of Ethics II

Individuals shall honor their responsibility to achieve and maintain the highest level of professional competence.

Rules of Ethics

A. Individuals shall engage in the provision of clinical services only when they hold the appropriate Certificate of Clinical Competence or when they are in the certification process and are supervised by an individual who holds the appropriate Certificate of Clinical Competence.

B. Individuals shall engage in only those aspects of the professions that are within the scope of their competence, considering their level of education, training, and experience.

C. Individuals shall continue their professional development throughout their careers.

D. Individuals shall delegate the provision of clinical services only to persons who are certified or to persons in the education or certification process who are appropriately supervised. The provision of support services may be delegated to persons who are neither certified nor in the certification process only when a certificate holder provides appropriate supervision.

E. Individuals shall prohibit any of their professional staff from providing services that exceed the staff member's competence, considering the staff member's level of education, training, and experience.

F. Individuals shall ensure that all equipment used in the provision of services is in proper working order and is properly calibrated.

Principle of Ethics III

Individuals shall honor their responsibility to the public by promoting public understanding of the professions, by supporting the development of services designed to fulfill the unmet needs of the public, and by providing accurate information in all communications involving any aspect of the professions.

Rules of Ethics

A. Individuals shall not misrepresent their credentials, competence, education, training, or experience.

B. Individuals shall not participate in professional activities that constitute a conflict of interest.

C. Individuals shall not misrepresent diagnostic information, services rendered, or products dispensed or engage in any scheme or artifice to defraud in connection with obtaining payment or reimbursement for such services or products.

D. Individuals' statements to the public shall provide accurate information about the nature and management of communication disorders, about the professions, and about professional services.

E. Individuals' statements to the public—advertising, announcing, and marketing their professional services, reporting research results, and promoting product—shall adhere to prevailing professional standards and shall not contain misrepresentations.

Principle of Ethics IV

Individuals shall honor their responsibilities to the professions and their relationships with colleagues, students, and members of allied professions. Individuals shall uphold the dignity and autonomy of the professions, maintain harmonious interprofessional and intraprofessional relationships, and accept the professions' self-imposed standards.

Rules of Ethics

A. Individuals shall prohibit anyone under their supervision from engaging in any practice that violates the Code of Ethics.

B. Individuals shall not engage in dishonesty, fraud, deceit, misrepresentation, or any form of conduct that adversely reflects on the professions or on the individual's fitness to serve persons professionally.

C. Individuals shall assign credit only to those who have contributed to a publication, presentation, or product. Credit shall be assigned in proportion to the contribution and only with the contributor's consent.

D. Individuals' statements to colleagues about professional services, research results, and products shall adhere to prevailing professional standards and shall contain no misrepresentations.

E. Individuals shall not provide professional services without exercising independent professional judgment, regardless of referral source or prescription.

F. Individuals shall not discriminate in their relationships with colleagues, students, and members of allied professions on the basis of race or ethnicity, gender, age, religion, national origin, sexual orientation, or disability.

G. Individuals who have reason to believe that the Code of Ethics has been violated shall inform the Ethical Practice Board.

H. Individuals shall cooperate fully with the Ethical Practice Board in its investigation and adjudication of matters related to this Code of Ethics.

Last revised January 1, 1994

Reprinted with permission from American Speech-Language-Hearing Association (1994). Code of ethics. ASHA, 36 (March, Suppl. 13), 1-2.

B

Excerpts from Sample Licensure Laws

EXCERPT FROM THE FLORIDA OT PRACTICE ACT, FL STAT § 468.217

468.217 Denial of or Refusal to Renew License; Suspension and Revocation of License and Other Disciplinary Measures

(1) The board may deny or refuse to renew a license, suspend or revoke a license, issue a reprimand, impose a fine, or impose probationary conditions upon a licensee, when the licensee or applicant for license has been guilty of unprofessional conduct which has endangered, or is likely to endanger, the health, welfare, or safety of the public. Such unprofessional conduct includes:

(a) Attempting to obtain, obtaining, or renewing a license to practice occupational therapy by bribery, by fraudulent misrepresentation, or through an error of the department or the board.

(b) Having a license to practice occupational therapy revoked, suspended, or otherwise acted against, including the denial of licensure, by the licensing authority of another state, territory, or country.

(c) Being convicted or found guilty, regardless of adjudication, of a crime in any jurisdiction which directly relates to the practice of occupational therapy or to the ability to practice occupational therapy. A plea of nolo contendere shall be considered a conviction for the purposes of this part.

(d) False, deceptive, or misleading advertising.

(e) Advertising, practicing, or attempting to practice under a name other than one's own name.

(f) Failing to report to the department any person who the licensee knows is in violation of this part or of the rules of the department or of the board.

(g) Aiding, assisting, procuring, or advising any unlicensed person to practice occupational therapy contrary to this part or to a rule of the department or the board.

(h) Failing to perform any statutory or legal obligation placed upon a licensed occupational therapist or occupational therapy assistant.

(i) Making or filing a report which the licensee knows to be false, intentionally or negligently failing to file a report or record required by state or federal law, willfully impeding or obstructing such filing or inducing another person to do so. Such reports or records include only those which are signed in the capacity as a licensed occupational therapist or occupational therapy assistant.

(j) Paying or receiving any commission, bonus,

kickback, or rebate to or from, or engaging in any split-fee arrangement in any form whatsoever with, a physician, organization, agency, or person, either directly or indirectly, for patients referred to providers of health care goods and services, including, but not limited to, hospitals, nursing homes, clinical laboratories, ambulatory surgical centers, or pharmacies. The provisions of this paragraph shall not be construed to prevent an occupational therapist or occupational therapy assistant from receiving a fee for professional consultation services.

(k) Exercising influence within a patient-therapist relationship for purposes of engaging a patient in sexual activity. A patient is presumed to be incapable of giving free, full, and informed consent to sexual activity with the patient's occupational therapist or occupational therapy assistant.

(l) Making deceptive, untrue, or fraudulent representations in the practice of occupational therapy or employing a trick or scheme in the practice of occupational therapy if such scheme or trick fails to conform to the generally prevailing standards of treatment in the occupational therapy community.

(m) Soliciting patients, either personally or through an agent, through the use of fraud, intimidation, undue influence, or a form of overreaching or vexatious conduct. A "solicitation" is any communication which directly or implicitly requests an immediate oral response from the recipient.

(n) Failing to keep written records justifying the course of treatment of the patient, including, but not limited to, patient histories, examination results, and test results.

(o) Exercising influence on the patient or client in such a manner as to exploit the patient or client for financial gain of the licensee or of a third party which includes, but is not limited to, the promoting or selling of services, goods, appliances, or drugs.

(p) Performing professional services which have not been duly authorized by the patient or client, or his or her legal representative, except as provided in s. 768.13.

(q) Gross or repeated malpractice or the failure to practice occupational therapy with that level of care, skill, and treatment which is recognized by a reasonably prudent similar occupational therapist or occupational therapy assistant as being acceptable under similar conditions and circumstances.

(r) Performing any procedure which, by the prevailing standards of occupational therapy practice in the community, would constitute experimentation on a human subject without first obtaining full, informed, and written consent.

(s) Practicing or offering to practice beyond the scope permitted by law or accepting and performing professional responsibilities which the licensee knows or has reason to know that he or she is not competent to perform.

(t) Being unable to practice occupational therapy with reasonable skill and safety to patients by reason of illness or use of alcohol, drugs, narcotics, chemicals, or any other type of material or as a result of any mental or physical condition. In enforcing this paragraph, the department shall have, upon probable cause, authority to compel an occupational therapist or occupational therapy assistant to submit to a mental or physical examination by physicians designated by the department. The failure of an occupational therapist or occupational therapy assistant to submit to such examination when so directed constitutes an admission of the allegations against him or her, upon which a default and final order may be entered without the taking of testimony or presentation of evidence, unless the failure was due to circumstances beyond his or her control. An occupational therapist or occupational therapy assistant affected under this paragraph shall at reasonable intervals be afforded an opportunity to demonstrate that he or she can resume the competent practice of occupational therapy with reasonable skill and safety to patients. In any proceeding under this paragraph, neither the record of proceedings nor the orders entered by the board shall be used against an occupational therapist or occupational therapy assistant in any other proceeding.

(u) Delegating professional responsibilities to a person when the licensee who is delegating such responsibilities knows or has reason to know that such person is not qualified by training, experience, or licensure to perform them.

(v) Violating any provision of this part, a rule of the board or department, or a lawful order of the board or department previously entered in a disciplinary hearing or failing to comply with a lawfully issued subpoena of the department.

(w) Conspiring with another licensee or with any other person to commit an act, or committing an act, which would tend to coerce, intimidate, or preclude another licensee from lawfully advertising his or her services.

(2) The board may not reinstate the license of an occupational therapist or occupational therapy assistant, or cause a license to be issued to a person it has deemed unqualified, until such time as the board is satisfied that such person has complied with all the terms and conditions set forth in the final order and is capable of safely engaging in the practice of occupational therapy.

History-s. 11, ch. 75-179; s. 36, ch. 78-95; s. 2, ch. 81-318; ss. 7, 12, 13, ch. 84-4; s. 4, ch. 91-429; s. 280, ch. 97-103.

EXCERPT FROM THE OT PRACTICE ACT, FL STAT § 458.223

468.223 Prohibitions; Penalties

(1) A person may not:

(a) Practice occupational therapy unless such person is licensed pursuant to ss. 468.201-468.225;

(b) Use, in connection with his or her name or place of business, the words "occupational therapist," "licensed occupational therapist," "occupational therapist registered," "occupational therapy assistant," "licensed occupational therapy assistant," "certified occupational therapy assistant"; the letters "OT," "LOT," "OTR," "OTA," "LOTA," or "COTA"; or any other words, letters, abbreviations, or insignia indicating or implying that he or she is an occupational therapist or an occupational therapy assistant or, in any way, orally or in writing, in print or by sign, directly or by implication, to represent himself or herself as an occupational therapist or an occupational therapy assistant unless the person is a holder of a valid license issued pursuant to ss. 468.201-468.225;

(c) Present as his or her own the license of another;

(d) Knowingly give false or forged evidence to the board or a member thereof;

(e) Use or attempt to use a license which has been suspended, revoked, or placed on inactive or delinquent status;

(f) Employ unlicensed persons to engage in the practice of occupational therapy; or

(g) Conceal information relative to any violation of ss. 468.201-468.225.

(2) Any person who violates any provision of this section commits a misdemeanor of the second degree, punishable as provided in s. 775.082 or s. 775.083.

History-s. 14, ch. 75-179; s. 2, ch. 81-318; ss. 10, 12, 13, ch. 84-4; s. 3, ch. 90-22; s. 4, ch. 91-429; s. 196, ch. 94-119; s. 281, ch. 97-103.

EXCERPT FROM THE PT PRACTICE ACT, FL STAT § 486.123

486.123 Sexual Misconduct in the Practice of Physical Therapy

The physical therapist-patient relationship is founded on mutual trust. Sexual misconduct in the practice of physical therapy means violation of the physical therapist-patient relationship through which the physical therapist uses that relationship to induce or attempt to induce the patient to engage, or to engage or attempt to engage the patient, in sexual activity outside the scope of practice or the scope of generally accepted examination or treatment of the patient. Sexual misconduct in the practice of physical therapy is prohibited.

EXCERPT FROM THE PT PRACTICE ACT, FL STAT § 486.125

486.125 Refusal, Revocation, or Suspension of License; Administrative Fines and Other Disciplinary Measures

(1) The following acts shall constitute grounds for which the disciplinary actions specified in subsection (2) may be taken:

(a) Being unable to practice physical therapy with reasonable skill and safety to patients by reason of illness or use of alcohol, drugs, narcotics, chemicals, or any other type of material or as a result of any mental or physical condition.

1. In enforcing this paragraph, upon a finding of the secretary or the secretary's designee that probable cause exists to believe that the licensee is unable to practice physical therapy due to the reasons stated in this paragraph, the department shall have the authority to compel a physical therapist or physical therapist assistant to submit to a mental or physical examination by a physician designated by the department. If the licensee refuses to comply with such order, the department's order directing such examination may be enforced by filing a petition for enforcement in the circuit court where the licensee resides or serves as a physical therapy practitioner. The licensee against whom the petition is filed shall not be named or identified by initials in any public court records or documents, and the proceedings shall be closed to the public. The department shall be entitled to the summary procedure provided in s. 51.011.

2. A physical therapist or physical therapist assistant whose license is suspended or revoked pursuant to this subsection shall, at reasonable intervals, be given an opportunity to demonstrate that she or he can resume the competent practice of physical therapy with reasonable skill and safety to patients.

3. Neither the record of proceeding nor the orders entered by the board in any proceeding under this subsection may be used against a physical therapist or physical therapist assistant in any other proceeding.

(b) Having committed fraud in the practice of physical therapy or deceit in obtaining a license as a physical therapist or as a physical therapist assistant.

(c) Being convicted or found guilty regardless of adjudication, of a crime in any jurisdiction which directly relates to the practice of physical therapy or to the ability to practice physical therapy. The entry of any plea of nolo contendere shall be considered a conviction for purpose of this chapter.

(d) Having treated or undertaken to treat human ailments by means other than by physical therapy, as defined in this chapter.

(e) Failing to maintain acceptable standards of physical therapy practice as set forth by the board in rules adopted pursuant to this chapter.

(f) Engaging directly or indirectly in the dividing, transferring, assigning, rebating, or refunding of fees received for professional services, or having been found to profit by means of a credit or other valuable consideration, such as an unearned commission, discount, or gratuity, with any person referring a patient or with any relative or business associate of the referring person. Nothing in this chapter shall be construed to prohibit the members of any regularly and properly organized business entity which is comprised of physical therapists and which is recognized under the laws of this state from making any division of their total fees among themselves as they determine necessary.

(g) Having a license revoked or suspended; having had other disciplinary action taken against her or him; or having had her or his application for a license refused, revoked, or suspended by the licensing authority of another state, territory, or country.

(h) Violating any provision of this chapter, a rule of the board or department, or a lawful order of the board or department previously entered in a disciplinary hearing.

(i) Making or filing a report or record which the licensee knows to be false. Such reports or records shall include only those which are signed in the capacity of a physical therapist.

(j) Practicing or offering to practice beyond the scope permitted by law or accepting and performing professional responsibilities which the licensee knows or has reason to know that she or he is not competent to perform, including, but not limited to, specific spinal manipulation.

(2) When the board finds any person guilty of any of the grounds set forth in subsection (1), it may enter an order imposing one or more of the following penalties:

(a) Refusal to certify to the department an application for licensure.

(b) Revocation or suspension of a license.

(c) Restriction of practice.

(d) Imposition of an administrative fine not to exceed $1,000 for each count or separate offense.

(e) Issuance of a reprimand.

(f) Placement of the physical therapist or physical therapist assistant on probation for a period of time and subject to such conditions as the board may specify, including, but not limited to, requiring the physical therapist or physical therapist assistant to submit to treatment, to attend continuing education courses, to submit to reexamination, or to work under the supervision of another physical therapist.

(g) Recovery of actual costs of investigation and prosecution.

(3) The board shall not reinstate the license of a physical therapist or physical therapist assistant or cause a license to be issued to a person it has deemed unqualified until such time as it is satisfied that she or he has complied with all the terms and conditions set forth in the final order and that such person is capable of safely engaging in the practice of physical therapy.

EXCERPT FROM THE PT PRACTICE ACT, FL STAT § 486.135

486.135 False Representation of Licensure, or Willful Misrepresentation or Fraudulent Representation to Obtain License, Unlawful

(1)

(a) It is unlawful for any person who is not licensed under this chapter as a physical therapist, or whose license has been suspended or revoked, to use in connection with her or his name or place of business the words "physical therapist," "physiotherapist," "physical therapy," "physiotherapy," "registered physical therapist," or "licensed physical therapist"; or the letters "PT," "PhT," "RPT," or "LPT"; or any other words, letters, abbreviations, or insignia indicating or implying that she or he is a physical therapist or to represent herself or himself as a physical therapist in any other way, orally, in writing, in print, or by sign, directly or by implication, unless physical therapy services are provided or supplied by a physical therapist licensed in accordance with this chapter.

(b) It is unlawful for any person who is not licensed under this chapter as a physical therapist assistant, or whose license has been suspended or revoked, to use in connection with her or his name

the words "physical therapist assistant," "licensed physical therapist assistant," "registered physical therapist assistant," or "physical therapy technician"; or the letters "PTA," "LPTA," "RPTA," or "PTT"; or any other words, letters, abbreviations, or insignia indicating or implying that she or he is a physical therapist assistant or to represent herself or himself as a physical therapist assistant in any other way, orally, in writing, in print, or by sign, directly or by implication.

(2) It is unlawful for any person to obtain or attempt to obtain a license under this chapter by any willful misrepresentation or any fraudulent representation.

EXCERPTS FROM THE FLORIDA SPEECH PATHOLOGY PRACTICE ACT, FL STAT § 468

468.1285 Prohibitions; Penalties

(1) No person shall knowingly:

(a) Practice speech-language pathology or audiology, unless the person is licensed pursuant to this part.

(b) Use terms such as, but not limited to: "speech pathologist," "speech therapy," "speech therapist," "speech correction," "speech correctionist," "speech clinic," "speech clinician," "language pathology," "language pathologist," "voice therapist," "voice pathology," "voice pathologist," "logopedics," "logopedist," "communicology," "communicologist," "cognitive communication therapy," "cognitive communication therapist," "aphasiologist," or "phoniatrist," or any title, designation, words, letters, abbreviations, or device tending to indicate that such person holds an active license as a speech-language pathologist when the person is not licensed as a speech-language pathologist pursuant to this part.

(c) Use terms such as, but not limited to: "audiology," "audiologist," "audiometrist," "audiological," "hearing therapy," "hearing therapist," "hearing clinic," "hearing clinician," "hearing aid audiologist," "aural habilitationalist," "aural rehabilitationalist," or any title, designation, words, letters, abbreviations, or device tending to indicate that such person holds an active license as an audiologist when the person is not licensed as an audiologist pursuant to this part.

(d) Present as his or her own the license of another.

(e) Use or attempt to use a license to practice speech-language pathology or audiology which has been suspended, revoked, or placed on inactive or delinquent status.

(f) Give false or forged evidence to the board or a member thereof.

(g) Employ unlicensed persons in the practice of speech-language pathology or audiology.

(h) Sell or fraudulently obtain or furnish any speech-language pathology or audiology diploma, license, or record of registration, or aid or abet in the same.

(i) Conceal information relative to violations of this part.

(2) Any person who is convicted of a violation of this section commits a misdemeanor of the second degree, punishable as provided in s. 775.082 or s. 775.083.

Disciplinary Proceedings

(1) The following acts constitute grounds for both disciplinary actions as set forth in subsection (2) and cease and desist or other related actions by the department as set forth in s. 455.228:

(a) Procuring or attempting to procure a license by bribery, by fraudulent misrepresentation, or through an error of the department or the board.

(b) Having a license revoked, suspended, or otherwise acted against, including denial of licensure, by the licensing authority of another state, territory, or country.

(c) Being convicted or found guilty of, or entering a plea of nolo contendere to, regardless of adjudication, a crime in any jurisdiction which directly relates to the practice of speech-language pathology or audiology.

(d) Making or filing a report or record which the licensee knows to be false, intentionally or negligently failing to file a report or records required by state or federal law, willfully impeding or obstructing such filing, or inducing another person to impede or obstruct such filing. Such report or record shall include only those reports or records which are

signed in one's capacity as a licensed speech-language pathologist or audiologist.

(e) Advertising goods or services in a manner which is fraudulent, false, deceptive, or misleading in form or content.

(f) Being proven guilty of fraud or deceit or of negligence, incompetency, or misconduct in the practice of speech-language pathology or audiology.

(g) Violating a lawful order of the board or department previously entered in a disciplinary hearing, or failing to comply with a lawfully issued subpoena of the board or department.

(h) Practicing with a revoked, suspended, inactive, or delinquent license.

(i) Using, or causing or promoting the use of, any advertising matter, promotional literature, testimonial, guarantee, warranty, label, brand, insignia, or other representation, however disseminated or published, which is misleading, deceiving, or untruthful.

(j) Showing or demonstrating or, in the event of sale, delivery of a product unusable or impractical for the purpose represented or implied by such action.

(k) Failing to submit to the board on an annual basis, or such other basis as may be provided by rule, certification of testing and calibration of such equipment as designated by the board and on the form approved by the board.

(l) Aiding, assisting, procuring, employing, or advising any licensee or business entity to practice speech-language pathology or audiology contrary to this part, chapter 455, or any rule adopted pursuant thereto.

(m) Violating any provision of this part or chapter 455 or any rule adopted pursuant thereto.

(n) Misrepresenting the professional services available in the fitting, sale, adjustment, service, or repair of a hearing aid, or using any other term or title which might connote the availability of professional services when such use is not accurate.

(o) Representing, advertising, or implying that a hearing aid or its repair is guaranteed without providing full disclosure of the identity of the guarantor; the nature, extent, and duration of the guarantee; and the existence of conditions or limitations imposed upon the guarantee.

(p) Representing, directly or by implication, that

a hearing aid utilizing bone conduction has certain specified features, such as the absence of anything in the ear or leading to the ear, or the like, without disclosing clearly and conspicuously that the instrument operates on the bone conduction principle and that in many cases of hearing loss this type of instrument may not be suitable.

(q) Stating or implying that the use of any hearing aid will improve or preserve hearing or prevent or retard the progression of a hearing impairment or that it will have any similar or opposite effect.

(r) Making any statement regarding the cure of the cause of a hearing impairment by the use of a hearing aid.

(s) Representing or implying that a hearing aid is or will be "custom-made," "made to order," or "prescription-made," or in any other sense specially fabricated for an individual, when such is not the case.

(t) Canvassing from house to house or by telephone, either in person or by an agent, for the purpose of selling a hearing aid, except that contacting persons who have evidenced an interest in hearing aids, or have been referred as in need of hearing aids, shall not be considered canvassing.

(u) Failing to notify the department in writing of a change in current mailing and place-of-practice address within 30 days after such change.

(v) Failing to provide all information as described in ss. 468.1225(5)(b), 468.1245(1), and 468.1246.

(w) Exercising influence on a client in such a manner as to exploit the client for financial gain of the licensee or of a third party.

(x) Practicing or offering to practice beyond the scope permitted by law or accepting and performing professional responsibilities the licensee or certificate holder knows, or has reason to know, the licensee or certificate holder is not competent to perform.

(y) Aiding, assisting, procuring, or employing any unlicensed person to practice speech-language pathology or audiology.

(z) Delegating or contracting for the performance of professional responsibilities by a person when the licensee delegating or contracting for performance of such responsibilities knows, or has reason to know, such person is not qualified by training, experience, and authorization to perform them.

(aa) Committing any act upon a patient or client which would constitute sexual battery or which would constitute sexual misconduct as defined pursuant to s. 468.1296.

(bb) Being unable to practice the profession for which he or she is licensed or certified under this chapter with reasonable skill or competence as a result of any mental or physical condition or by reason of illness, drunkenness, or use of drugs, narcotics, chemicals, or any other substance. In enforcing this paragraph, upon a finding by the secretary, his or her designee, or the board that probable cause exists to believe that the licensee or certificate holder is unable to practice the profession because of the reasons stated in this paragraph, the department shall have the authority to compel a licensee or certificate holder to submit to a mental or physical examination by a physician, psychologist, clinical social worker, marriage and family therapist, or mental health counselor designated by the department or board. If the licensee or certificate holder refuses to comply with the department's order directing the examination, such order may be enforced by filing a petition for enforcement in the circuit court in the circuit in which the licensee or certificate holder resides or does business. The department shall be entitled to the summary procedure provided in s. 51.011. A licensee or certificate holder affected under this paragraph shall at reasonable intervals be afforded an opportunity to demonstrate that he or she can resume the competent practice for which he or she is licensed or certified with reasonable skill and safety to patients.

(2) When the board finds any person guilty of any of the acts set forth in subsection (1), it may issue an order imposing one or more of the following penalties:

(a) Refusal to certify, or to certify with restrictions, an application for licensure.

(b) Suspension or permanent revocation of a license.

(c) Issuance of a reprimand.

(d) Restriction of the authorized scope of practice.

(e) Imposition of an administrative fine not to exceed $1,000 for each count or separate offense.

(f) Placement of the licensee or certificate holder on probation for a period of time and subject to such conditions as the board may specify. Those conditions may include, but are not limited to, requiring the licensee or certificate holder to undergo treatment, attend continuing education courses, submit to be reexamined, work under the supervision of another licensee, or satisfy any terms which are reasonably tailored to the violation found.

(g) Corrective action.

(3) The department shall reissue the license or certificate which has been suspended or revoked upon certification by the board that the licensee or certificate holder has complied with all of the terms and conditions set forth in the final order.

468.1296 Sexual Misconduct

Sexual misconduct by any person licensed or certified in the practice of his or her profession is prohibited. Sexual misconduct means to induce or to attempt to induce the patient to engage, or to engage or to attempt to engage the patient, in sexual activity outside the scope of practice or the scope of generally accepted examination or treatment of the patient.

C

Excerpts from the Prospective Payment Manual Including Rules in Relation to Group Treatment and Definition of Therapy Time

Medicare Provider Reimbursement Manual, Part 1
Department of Health and Human Services
Health Care Financing Administration
Excepted from the PPS Prospective Payment System Provider Manual
Transmittal No. 405 Date July 1998

2837. REPORTING REHABILITATIVE THERAPY MINUTES ON THE MDS FOR PURPOSES OF MEDICARE PAYMENT

In Section P of the MDS, the clinician records the number of days and minutes of rehabilitative therapy (PT, OT, ST) received by the individual beneficiary during the past 7 days, and in the case of the Medicare 5 day assessment, since admission to the SNF. The rehabilitative therapy time reported on the MDS is a record of the time the patient spent receiving therapy services, not a record of the therapist's time. As stated in the August 1996 publication, Long Term Care Resident Assessment Instrument Questions and Answers, Version 2.0, the patient's "therapy time starts when he begins the first treatment activity or task and ends when he finishes with the last apparatus and the treatment is ended." Set-up time is included, as is time under the therapist's or therapy assistant's direct supervision.

Whether the time spent evaluating the patient is counted depends on whether it is an initial evaluation or an evaluation performed after the course of therapy has begun. The time it takes to perform an initial evaluation and developing the treatment goals and the plan of care for the patient cannot be counted as minutes of therapy received by the patient. However, reevaluations that are performed once a therapy regimen is underway (e.g., evaluating goal achievement as part of the therapy session) may be counted as minutes of therapy received. This policy was established because we do not wish to give an incentive to perform initial evaluations for therapy services for patients who have no need of those specialized services. However, we believe that the initial assessment is an appropriate cost of doing business. Therefore, the cost of the initial assessment is included in the payment rates.

Likewise, throughout the course of treatment, the time it takes for the therapist to perform the required documentation may not be counted as time provided to the beneficiary.

Note: The example for counting therapy time on page 3-170 of the Long Term Care Resident Assessment Instrument User's Manual, Version 2.0 is incorrect. Cross out that example. A new example will be included in the revised version.

The Long Term Care Resident Assessment Instrument Questions and Answers, Version 2.0 also clarifies how to account for therapy provided to an individual within a group setting. It states that if the group has four or fewer participants per supervising therapist (or therapy assistant) then it is appropriate to report the full time as therapy for each patient. The example used is that of a therapist working with three patients for 45 minutes on training to return to the community. Each patient's MDS would reflect receipt of 45 minutes of therapy for this session.

Although we recognize that receiving physical, occupational or speech therapy as part of a group has clinical merit in select situations, we do not believe that services received within a group setting should account for more than 25 percent of the Medicare patient's therapy regimen during his SNF stay. For this reason, no more than 25 percent of the minutes reported in Section P may be provided within a group setting. To summarize: the minutes of therapy provided by at least one supervising therapist (or therapy assistant) within a group of 4 or fewer participants, may be fully counted, provided that those minutes account for no more than 25 percent of the patient's weekly therapy as reported in section P of the MDS. The supervising therapist may not be supervising any individuals other than the 4 or fewer individuals who are in the group at the time of the therapy session. Group therapy time in excess of the 25 percent threshold cannot be counted.

In addition, all therapy services must meet each of the following criteria in order to be coded on the MDS as rehabilitative therapy:

- The service must be ordered by a physician.
- The therapy intervention must be based on a qualified therapist's evaluation and plan of care as documented in the resident's record.
- An appropriate licensed or certified individual must provide or directly supervise the therapeutic service and coordinate the intervention with nursing service.

Reporting minutes of therapy in Section T is somewhat different. Section T must be completed with each Medicare PPS assessment, but in the case of a Medicare 5 day assessment, the clinician captures minutes of therapy that are anticipated for the patient during the first 15 days of his nursing home stay. This makes it possible for the patient to classify into the appropriate RUG rehabilitation group based on his anticipated receipt of rehabilitative therapy when the assessment is done during the first few

days of the SNF stay and there has not been enough time to provide more than the beginning of a course of rehabilitative therapy. The RUG grouper takes into consideration both the days and minutes already received by the patient as reported in Section P and the days and minutes expected to be received in the first 15 days of the stay. The number of days and minutes expected, as reported in section T should include those already received. For example, if the patient received an hour of therapy on both the fourth and fifth days (a Monday and Tuesday) of his SNF stay and the prescribed regimen is for him to receive an hour of therapy daily, Monday through Friday, during his first 2 weeks in the SNF; 2 days and 120 minutes would be reported in Section P, and 10 days and 600 minutes would be reported in Section T. The 10 days and 600 minutes includes the 2 days and 120 minutes already received plus the upcoming 3 days and 180 minutes in the first week and the 5 days and 300 minutes of therapy in the second week.

The directions for completion of Section P instruct the assessor to look back over the "last 7 calendar days," counting only post admission days and minutes of therapy, when counting the days and minutes of rehabilitation therapy administered. Seven calendar days are, by definition, consecutive days. In the case of a Medicare 5 day assessment, however, the assessor will choose as the assessment reference date (MDS item A3a) any day 1-8 of the stay, and will look back over the last 7 calendar days (or over the days since admission if the assessment reference date is earlier than day 7) and count the number of days upon which more than 15 minutes of therapy were administered, and will count the number of minutes that were provided to the individual patient during those days.

It is irrelevant if there is a break in therapy for a weekend or holiday during that time. For example, if day 5 of the stay is chosen as the assessment reference date, the assessor would look back to admission to count the patient's OT, PT, and ST time. If PT was provided for 50 minutes on both the second and fifth days of the stay, that would be recorded as 2 days of PT and 100 minutes of PT. The actual time that therapy was provided should be recorded. It does NOT have to be expressed in multiples of 15 or 10.

Further clarification of Section T:

(1) In order to complete the last part of Section T, item 3, 'Case Mix Group' put the three digit char-

acter code for the RUG group into the first 3 spaces of the 5 space Medicare case-mix item and '07' into the last 2 spaces. For example, a patient who classifies into the least intensive Clinically Complex group would be coded in item T3 (Medicare case-mix) as "CA107" in the Medicare blocks. Instructions for completion of the State blocks will be issued to providers by their States.

(2) Physical, speech and occupational therapy provided outside the facility IS captured in Section T, as long as the staff providing therapy meet the qualifiers. See SOM Transmittal #272, pp. R64, "The therapy treatment may occur inside or outside the facility."

(3) Pay attention to the skip instructions for item T2 in italics at the top of the item. Be sure you are using the MDS 2.0, 1/30/98 version.

(4) The items at T2a-e capture information based on the same episode when the resident walked the farthest without sitting down, regardless of the need for assistance to get to a standing position. This episode may be a time during therapy. This observation item captures the single HIGHEST level of independence in the observation period (in contrast to capturing the most assistance needed in the observation period, as in Section G of the MDS).

Since this most independent episode may have occurred in therapy (even if the patient was using parallel bars at the time) or on the nursing unit, the communication between therapists and nursing staff ON ALL SHIFTS is essential.

(5) Section T1b of the MDS, the item in which expected therapy is reported, may only be completed for the 5 day Medicare required assessment or on a Medicare readmission/return assessment (AA8b = 1 or 5).

(6) If your MDS automation software incorrectly requires that MDS item T1b, c and d be addressed on the Initial Admission Assessment (AA8a = 01), then the following "work-around" can be used until the software is corrected:

Enter "0" at MDS item T1b. This will allow MDS items T1c and d to be skipped. One validation error will occur indicating that T1b should be skipped. This error can be ignored until the software is corrected. Note that if this work-around is not used, the facility will receive 3 error messages (one for each MDS item T1b, c, and d).

D

Federal Statutes Pertaining to Medicare and Medicaid Fraud

18 USCA § 287

United States Code Annotated
Title 18. Crimes and Criminal Procedure
Part I-Crimes
Chapter 15-Claims and Services in Matters Affecting Government

§ 287 False, Fictitious or Fraudulent Claims

Whoever makes or presents to any person or officer in the civil, military, or naval service of the United States, or to any department or agency thereof, any claim upon or against the United States, or any department or agency thereof, knowing such claim to be false, fictitious, or fraudulent, shall be imprisoned not more than five years and shall be subject to a fine in the amount provided in this title.

18 USCA § 1001

United States Code Annotated
Title 18. Crimes and Criminal Procedure
Part I-Crimes
Chapter 47-Fraud and False Statements

§ 1001 Statements or Entries Generally

(a) Except as otherwise provided in this section, whoever, in any matter within the jurisdiction of the executive, legislative, or judicial branch of the Government of the United States, knowingly and willfully-

(1) falsifies, conceals, or covers up by any trick, scheme, or device a material fact;

(2) makes any materially false, fictitious, or fraudulent statement or representation; or

(3) makes or uses any false writing or document knowing the same to contain any materially false, fictitious, or fraudulent statement or entry;

shall be fined under this title or imprisoned not more than 5 years, or both.

(b) Subsection (a) does not apply to a party to a judicial proceeding, or that party's counsel, for statements, representations, writings or documents submitted by such party or counsel to a judge or magistrate in that proceeding.

(c) With respect to any matter within the jurisdiction of the legislative branch, subsection (a) shall apply only to-

(1) administrative matters, including a claim for

payment, a matter related to the procurement of property or services, personnel or employment practices, or support services, or a document required by law, rule, or regulation to be submitted to the Congress or any office or officer within the legislative branch; or

(2) any investigation or review, conducted pursuant to the authority of any committee, subcommittee, commission or office of the Congress, consistent with applicable rules of the House or Senate.

18 USCA § 1341

United States Code Annotated
Title 18. Crimes and Criminal Procedure
Part I-Crimes
Chapter 63-Mail Fraud

§ 1341 Frauds and Swindles

Whoever, having devised or intending to devise any scheme or artifice to defraud, or for obtaining money or property by means of false or fraudulent pretenses, representations, or promises, or to sell, dispose of, loan, exchange, alter, give away, distribute, supply, or furnish or procure for unlawful use any counterfeit or spurious coin, obligation, security, or other article, or anything represented to be or intimated or held out to be such counterfeit or spurious article, for the purpose of executing such scheme or artifice or attempting so to do, places in any post office or authorized depository for mail matter, any matter or thing whatever to be sent or delivered by the Postal Service, or deposits or causes to be deposited any matter or thing whatever to be sent or delivered by any private or commercial interstate carrier, or takes or receives therefrom, any such matter or thing, or knowingly causes to be delivered by mail or such carrier according to the direction thereon, or at the place at which it is directed to be delivered by the person to whom it is addressed, any such matter or thing, shall be fined under this title or imprisoned not more than five years, or both. If the violation affects a financial institution, such person shall be fined not more than $1,000,000 or imprisoned not more than 30 years, or both.

18 USCA § 286

United States Code Annotated
Title 18. Crimes and Criminal Procedure
Part I-Crimes
Chapter 15-Claims and Services in Matters Affecting Government

§ 286 Conspiracy to Defraud the Government with Respect to Claims

Whoever enters into any agreement, combination, or conspiracy to defraud the United States, or any department or agency thereof, by obtaining or aiding to obtain the payment or allowance of any false, fictitious or fraudulent claim, shall be fined under this title or imprisoned not more than ten years, or both.

18 USCA § 371

United States Code Annotated
Title 18. Crimes and Criminal Procedure
Part I-Crimes
Chapter 19-Conspiracy

§ 371 Conspiracy to Commit Offense or to Defraud the United States

If two or more persons conspire either to commit any offense against the United States, or to defraud the United States, or any agency thereof in any manner or for any purpose, and one or more of such persons do any act to effect the object of the conspiracy, each shall be fined under this title or imprisoned not more than five years, or both.

If, however, the offense, the commission of which is the object of the conspiracy, is a misdemeanor only, the punishment for such conspiracy shall not exceed the maximum punishment provided for such misdemeanor.

18 USCA § 641

United States Code Annotated
Title 18. Crimes and Criminal Procedure
Part I-Crimes
Chapter 31-Embezzlement and Theft

§ 641 Public Money, Property or Records

Whoever embezzles, steals, purloins, or knowingly converts to his use or the use of another, or without authority, sells, conveys or disposes of any record, voucher, money, or thing of value of the United States or of any department or agency thereof, or any property made or being made under contract for the United States or any department or agency thereof; or

Whoever receives, conceals, or retains the same with intent to convert it to his use or gain, knowing it to have been embezzled, stolen, purloined or converted—

Shall be fined under this title or imprisoned not more than ten years, or both; but if the value of such property does not exceed the sum of $1,000, he shall be fined under this title or imprisoned not more than one year, or both.

The word "value" means face, par, or market value, or cost price, either wholesale or retail, whichever is greater.

18 USCA § 1343

United States Code Annotated
Title 18. Crimes and Criminal Procedure
Part I-Crimes
Chapter 63-Mail Fraud

§ 1343 Fraud by Wire, Radio, or Television

Whoever, having devised or intending to devise any scheme or artifice to defraud, or for obtaining money or property by means of false or fraudulent pretenses, representations, or promises, transmits or causes to be transmitted by means of wire, radio, or television communication in interstate or foreign commerce, any writings, signs, signals, pictures, or sounds for the purpose of executing such scheme or

artifice, shall be fined under this title or imprisoned not more than five years, or both. If the violation affects a financial institution, such person shall be fined not more than $1,000,000 or imprisoned not more than 30 years, or both.

18 USCA § 1956

United States Code Annotated
Title 18. Crimes and Criminal Procedure
Part I-Crimes
Chapter 95-Racketeering

§ 1956 Laundering of Monetary Instruments

(a)(1) Whoever, knowing that the property involved in a financial transaction represents the proceeds of some form of unlawful activity, conducts or attempts to conduct such a financial transaction which in fact involves the proceeds of specified unlawful activity-

(A)(i) with the intent to promote the carrying on of specified unlawful activity; or

(ii) with intent to engage in conduct constituting a violation of section 7201 or 7206 of the Internal Revenue Code of 1986; or

(B) knowing that the transaction is designed in whole or in part-

(i) to conceal or disguise the nature, the location, the source, the ownership, or the control of the proceeds of specified unlawful activity; or

(ii) to avoid a transaction reporting requirement under State or Federal law,

shall be sentenced to a fine of not more than $500,000 or twice the value of the property involved in the transaction, whichever is greater, or imprisonment for not more than twenty years, or both.

(2) Whoever transports, transmits, or transfers, or attempts to transport, transmit, or transfer a monetary instrument or funds from a place in the United States to or through a place outside the United States or to a place in the United States from or through a place outside the United States-

(A) with the intent to promote the carrying on of specified unlawful activity; or

(B) knowing that the monetary instrument or funds involved in the transportation, transmission, or transfer represent the proceeds of some form of unlawful activity and knowing that such transportation, transmission, or transfer is designed in whole or in part—

    (i) to conceal or disguise the nature, the location, the source, the ownership, or the control of the proceeds of specified unlawful activity; or

    (ii) to avoid a transaction reporting requirement under State or Federal law,

      shall be sentenced to a fine of not more than $500,000 or twice the value of the monetary instrument or funds involved in the transportation, transmission, or transfer whichever is greater, or imprisonment for not more than twenty years, or both. For the purpose of the offense described in subparagraph (B), the defendant's knowledge may be established by proof that a law enforcement officer represented the matter specified in subparagraph (B) as true, and the defendant's subsequent statements or actions indicate that the defendant believed such representations to be true.

(3) Whoever, with the intent-

(A) to promote the carrying on of specified unlawful activity;

(B) to conceal or disguise the nature, location, source, ownership, or control of property believed to be the proceeds of specified unlawful activity; or

(C) to avoid a transaction reporting requirement under State or Federal law,

conducts or attempts to conduct a financial transaction involving property represented to be the proceeds of specified unlawful activity, or property used to conduct or facilitate specified unlawful activity, shall be fined under this title or imprisoned for not more than 20 years, or both. For purposes of this paragraph and paragraph (2), the term "represented" means any representation made by a law enforcement officer or by another person at the direction of, or with the approval of, a Federal official authorized to investigate or prosecute violations of this section.

(b) Whoever conducts or attempts to conduct a transaction described in subsection (a)(1) or (a)(3), or a transportation, transmission, or transfer described in subsection (a)(2), is liable to the United States for a civil penalty of not more than the greater of—

(1) the value of the property, funds, or monetary instruments involved in the transaction; or

    (2) $10,000.

(c) As used in this section-

(1) the term "knowing that the property involved in a financial transaction represents the proceeds of some form of unlawful activity" means that the person knew the property involved in the transaction represented proceeds from some form, though not necessarily which form, of activity that constitutes a felony under State, Federal, or foreign law, regardless of whether or not such activity is specified in paragraph (7);

(2) the term "conducts" includes initiating, concluding, or participating in initiating, or concluding a transaction;

(3) the term "transaction" includes a purchase, sale, loan, pledge, gift, transfer, delivery, or other disposition, and with respect to a financial institution includes a deposit, withdrawal, transfer between accounts, exchange of currency, loan, extension of credit, purchase or sale of any stock, bond, certificate of deposit, or other monetary instrument, use of a safe deposit box, or any other payment, transfer, or delivery by, through, or to a financial institution, by whatever means effected;

(4) the term "financial transaction" means (A) a transaction which in any way or degree affects interstate or foreign commerce (i) involving the movement of funds by wire or other means or (ii) involving one or more monetary instruments, or (iii) involving the transfer of title to any real property, vehicle, vessel, or aircraft, or (B) a transaction involving the use of a financial institution which is engaged in, or the activities of which affect, interstate or foreign commerce in any way or degree;

(5) the term "monetary instruments" means (i) coin or currency of the United States or of any other country, travelers' checks, personal checks, bank checks, and money orders, or (ii) investment securities or negotiable instruments, in bearer form or otherwise in such form that title thereto passes upon delivery;

(6) the term "financial institution" has the definition given that term in section 5312(a)(2) of title 31, United States Code, or the regulations promulgated thereunder;

(7) the term "specified unlawful activity" means-

(A) any act or activity constituting an offense listed in section 1961(1) of this title except an act which is indictable under subchapter II of chapter 53 of title 31;

(B) with respect to a financial transaction occurring in whole or in part in the United States, an offense against a foreign nation involving-

(i) the manufacture, importation, sale, or distribution of a controlled substance (as such term is defined for the purposes of the Controlled Substances Act);

(ii) murder, kidnapping, robbery, extortion, or destruction of property by means of explosive or fire;

(iii) fraud, or any scheme or attempt to defraud, by or against a foreign bank (as defined in paragraph 7 of section 1(b) of the International Banking Act of 1978 [FN1]);

(C) any act or acts constituting a continuing criminal enterprise, as that term is defined in section 408 of the Controlled Substances Act (21 USC 848);

(D) an offense under section 32 (relating to the destruction of aircraft), section 37 (relating to violence at international airports), section 115 (relating to influencing, impeding, or retaliating against a Federal official by threatening or injuring a family member), section 152 (relating to concealment of assets; false oaths and claims; bribery), section 215 (relating to commissions or gifts for procuring loans), section 351 (relating to congressional or Cabinet officer assassination), any of sections 500 through 503 (relating to certain counterfeiting offenses), section 513 (relating to securities of States and private entities), section 542 (relating to entry of goods by means of false statements), section 545 (relating to smuggling goods into the United States), section 549 (relating to removing goods from Customs custody), section 641 (relating to public money, property, or records), section 656 (relating to theft, embezzlement, or misapplication by bank officer or employee), section 657 (relating to lending, credit, and insurance institutions), section 658 (relating to property mortgaged or pledged to farm credit agencies), section 666 (relating to theft or bribery concerning programs receiving Federal funds), section 793, 794, or 798 (relating to espionage), section 831 (relating to prohibited transactions involving nuclear materials), section 844(f) or (i) (relating to destruction by explosives or fire of Government property or property affecting interstate or foreign commerce), section 875 (relating to interstate communications), section 956 (relating to conspiracy to kill, kidnap, maim, or injure certain property in a foreign country), section 1005 (relating to fraudulent bank entries), 1006 (relating to fraudulent Federal credit institution entries), 1007 (relating to fraudulent Federal Deposit Insurance transactions), 1014 (relating to fraudulent loan or credit applications), 1032 (relating to concealment of assets from conservator, receiver, or liquidating agent of financial institution), section 1111 (relating to murder), section 1114 (relating to murder of United States law enforcement officials), section 1116 (relating to murder of foreign officials, official guests, or internationally protected persons), section 1201 (relating to kidnapping), section 1203 (relating to hostage taking), section 1361 (relating to willful injury of Government property), section 1363 (relating to destruction of property within the special maritime and territorial jurisdiction), section 1708 (theft from the mail), section 1751 (relating to Presidential assassination), section 2113 or 2114 (relating to bank and postal robbery and theft), section 2280 (relating to violence against maritime navigation), section 2281 (relating to violence against maritime fixed platforms), section 2319 (relating to copyright infringement), section 2320 (relating to trafficking in counterfeit goods and services), section 2332 (relating to terrorist acts abroad against United States nationals), section 2332a (relating to use of weapons of mass destruction), section 2332b (relating to international terrorist acts transcending national boundaries), or section 2339A (relating to providing material support to terrorists) of this title, section 46502 of title 49, United States Code, a felony violation of the Chemical Diversion and Trafficking Act of 1988 (relating to precursor and essential chemicals), section 590 of the Tariff Act of 1930 (19 USC 1590) (relating to aviation smuggling), section 422 of the Controlled Substances Act (relating to transportation of drug paraphernalia), section 38(c) (relating to criminal violations) of the Arms Export Control Act, section 11 (relating to violations) of the Export Administration Act of 1979, section 206 (relating to penalties) of the International Emergency Economic Powers Act, section 16 (relating to offenses and punishment) of the Trading with the Enemy Act, any felony violation of section 15 of the Food Stamp Act of 1977 (relating to food stamp fraud) involving a quantity of coupons having a value of not less than $5,000, or any felony violation of the Foreign Corrupt Practices Act; or

(E) a felony violation of the Federal Water Pollution Control Act (33 USC 1251 et seq.), the Ocean Dumping Act (33 USC 1401 et seq.), the Act to Prevent Pollution from Ships (33 USC 1901 et seq.), the Safe Drinking Water Act (42 USC 300f et seq.), or the Resources Conservation and Recovery Act (42 USC 6901 et seq.).

(F) Any act or activity constituting an offense involving a Federal health care offense.

(8) the term "State" includes a State of the United States, the District of Columbia, and any commonwealth, territory, or possession of the United States.

(d) Nothing in this section shall supersede any provision of Federal, State, or other law imposing criminal penalties or affording civil remedies in addition to those provided for in this section.

(e) Violations of this section may be investigated by such components of the Department of Justice as the Attorney General may direct, and by such components of the Department of the Treasury as the Secretary of the Treasury may direct, as appropriate and, with respect to offenses over which the United States Postal Service has jurisdiction, by the Postal Service. Such authority of the Secretary of the Treasury and the Postal Service shall be exercised in accordance with an agreement which shall be entered into by the Secretary of the Treasury, the Postal Service, and the Attorney General. Violations of this section involving offenses described in paragraph (c)(7)(E) may be investigated by such components of the Department of Justice as the Attorney General may direct, and the National Enforcement Investigations Center of the Environmental Protection Agency.

(f) There is extraterritorial jurisdiction over the conduct prohibited by this section if-

(1) the conduct is by a United States citizen or, in the case of a non-United States citizen, the conduct occurs in part in the United States; and

(2) the transaction or series of related transactions involves funds or monetary instruments of a value exceeding $10,000.

(g) Notice of conviction of financial institutions- If any financial institution or any officer, director, or employee of any financial institution has been found guilty of an offense under this section, section 1957 or 1960 of this title, or section 5322 or 5324 of title 31, the Attorney General shall provide written notice of such fact to the appropriate regulatory agency for the financial institution.

(h) Any person who conspires to commit any offense defined in this section or section 1957 shall be subject to the same penalties as those prescribed for the offense the commission of which was the object of the conspiracy.

18 USCA § 1957

United States Code Annotated
Title 18. Crimes and Criminal Procedure
Part I-Crimes
Chapter 95-Racketeering

§ 1957 Engaging in Monetary Transactions in Property Derived From Specified Unlawful Activity

(a) Whoever, in any of the circumstances set forth in subsection (d), knowingly engages or attempts to engage in a monetary transaction in criminally derived property that is of a value greater than $10,000 and is derived from specified unlawful activity, shall be punished as provided in subsection (b).

(b)(1) Except as provided in paragraph (2), the punishment for an offense under this section is a fine under title 18, United States Code, or imprisonment for not more than ten years or both.

(2) The court may impose an alternate fine to that imposable under paragraph (1) of not more than twice the amount of the criminally derived property involved in the transaction.

(c) In a prosecution for an offense under this section, the Government is not required to prove the defendant knew that the offense from which the criminally derived property was derived was specified unlawful activity.

(d) The circumstances referred to in subsection (a) are-

(1) that the offense under this section takes place in the United States or in the special maritime and territorial jurisdiction of the United States; or

(2) that the offense under this section takes place outside the United States and such special jurisdiction, but the defendant is a United States person (as defined in section 3077 of this title, but excluding the class described in paragraph (2)(D) of such section).

(e) Violations of this section may be investigated by such components of the Department of Justice as the Attorney General may direct, and by such components of the Department of the Treasury as the Secretary of the Treasury may direct, as appropriate and, with respect to offenses over which the United States Postal Service has jurisdiction, by the Postal Service. Such authority of the Secretary of the Treasury and the Postal Service shall be exercised in accordance with an agreement which shall be entered into by the Secretary of the Treasury, the Postal Service, and the Attorney General.

(f) As used in this section—

(1) the term "monetary transaction" means the deposit, withdrawal, transfer, or exchange, in or affecting interstate or foreign commerce, of funds or a monetary instrument (as defined in section 1956(c)(5) of this title) by, through, or to a financial institution (as defined in section 1956 of this title), including any transaction that would be a financial transaction under section 1956(c)(4)(B) of this title, but such term does not include any transaction necessary to preserve a person's right to representation as guaranteed by the sixth amendment to the Constitution;

(2) the term "criminally derived property" means any property constituting, or derived from, proceeds obtained from a criminal offense; and

(3) the term "specified unlawful activity" has the meaning given that term in section 1956 of this title.

18 USCA § 1961

United States Code Annotated
Title 18. Crimes and Criminal Procedure
Part I-Crimes
Chapter 96-Racketeer Influenced and Corrupt Organizations

§ 1961 Definitions

As used in this chapter—

(1) "racketeering activity" means (A) any act or threat involving murder, kidnapping, gambling, arson, robbery, bribery, extortion, dealing in obscene matter, or dealing in a controlled substance or listed chemical (as defined in section 102 of the Controlled Substances Act), which is chargeable under State law and punishable by imprisonment for more than one year; (B) any act which is indictable under any of the following provisions of title 18, United States Code: Section 201 (relating to bribery), section 224 (relating to sports bribery), sections 471, 472, and 473 (relating to counterfeiting), section 659 (relating to theft from interstate shipment) if the act indictable under section 659 is felonious, section 664 (relating to embezzlement from pension and welfare funds), sections 891-894 (relating to extortionate credit transactions), section 1028 (relating to fraud and related activity in connection with identification documents), section 1029 (relating to fraud and related activity in connection with access devices), section 1084 (relating to the transmission of gambling information), section 1341 (relating to mail fraud), section 1343 (relating to wire fraud), section 1344 (relating to financial institution fraud), section 1425 (relating to the procurement of citizenship or nationalization unlawfully), section 1426 (relating to the reproduction of naturalization or citizenship papers), section 1427 (relating to the sale of naturalization or citizenship papers), sections 1461-1465 (relating to obscene matter), section 1503 (relating to obstruction of justice), section 1510 (relating to obstruction of criminal investigations), section 1511 (relating to the obstruction of State or local law enforcement), section 1512 (relating to tampering with a witness, victim, or an informant), section 1513 (relating to retaliating against a witness, victim, or an informant), section 1542 (relating to false statement in application and use of passport), section 1543 (relating to forgery or false use of passport), section 1544 (relating to misuse of passport), section 1546 (relating to fraud and misuse of visas, permits, and other documents), sections 1581-1588 (relating to peonage and slavery), section 1951 (relating to interference with commerce, robbery, or extortion), section 1952 (relating to racketeering), section 1953 (relating to interstate transportation of wagering paraphernalia), section 1954 (relating to unlawful welfare fund payments), section 1955 (relating to the prohibition of illegal gambling businesses), section 1956 (relating to the laundering of monetary instruments), section 1957 (relating to engaging in monetary transactions in property derived from specified unlawful activity), section 1958 (relating to use of interstate commerce facilities in the commission of murder-for-hire), sections 2251, 2251A, 2252, and 2260 (relating to sexual exploitation of children), sections 2312 and 2313

(relating to interstate transportation of stolen motor vehicles), sections 2314 and 2315 (relating to interstate transportation of stolen property), section 2318 (relating to trafficking in counterfeit labels for phonorecords, computer programs or computer program documentation or packaging and copies of motion pictures or other audiovisual works), section 2319 (relating to criminal infringement of a copyright), section 2319A (relating to unauthorized fixation of and trafficking in sound recordings and music videos of live musical performances), section 2320 (relating to trafficking in goods or services bearing counterfeit marks), section 2321 (relating to trafficking in certain motor vehicles or motor vehicle parts), sections 2341-2346 (relating to trafficking in contraband cigarettes), sections 2421-24 (relating to white slave traffic), (C) any act which is indictable under title 29, United States Code, section 186 (dealing with restrictions on payments and loans to labor organizations) or section 501(c) (relating to embezzlement from union funds), (D) any offense involving fraud connected with a case under title 11 (except a case under section 157 of this title), fraud in the sale of securities, or the felonious manufacture, importation, receiving, concealment, buying, selling, or otherwise dealing in a controlled substance or listed chemical (as defined in section 102 of the Controlled Substances Act), punishable under any law of the United States, (E) any act which is indictable under the Currency and Foreign Transactions Reporting Act, or (F) any act which is indictable under the Immigration and Nationality Act, section 274 (relating to bringing in and harboring certain aliens), section 277 (relating to aiding or assisting certain aliens to enter the United States), or section 278 (relating to importation of alien for immoral purpose) if the act indictable under such section of such Act was committed for the purpose of financial gain;

(2) "State" means any State of the United States, the District of Columbia, the Commonwealth of Puerto Rico, any territory or possession of the United States, any political subdivision, or any department, agency, or instrumentality thereof;

(3) "person" includes any individual or entity capable of holding a legal or beneficial interest in property;

(4) "enterprise" includes any individual, partnership, corporation, association, or other legal entity, and any union or group of individuals associated in fact although not a legal entity;

(5) "pattern of racketeering activity" requires at least two acts of racketeering activity, one of which occurred after the effective date of this chapter and the last of which occurred within ten years (excluding any period of imprisonment) after the commission of a prior act of racketeering activity;

(6) "unlawful debt" means a debt (A) incurred or contracted in gambling activity which was in violation of the law of the United States, a State or political subdivision thereof, or which is unenforceable under State or Federal law in whole or in part as to principal or interest because of the laws relating to usury, and (B) which was incurred in connection with the business of gambling in violation of the law of the United States, a State or political subdivision thereof, or the business of lending money or a thing of value at a rate usurious under State or Federal law, where the usurious rate is at least twice the enforceable rate;

(7) "racketeering investigator" means any attorney or investigator so designated by the Attorney General and charged with the duty of enforcing or carrying into effect this chapter;

(8) "racketeering investigation" means any inquiry conducted by any racketeering investigator for the purpose of ascertaining whether any person has been involved in any violation of this chapter or of any final order, judgment, or decree of any court of the United States, duly entered in any case or proceeding arising under this chapter;

(9) "documentary material" includes any book, paper, document, record, recording, or other material; and

(10) "Attorney General" includes the Attorney General of the United States, the Deputy Attorney General of the United States, the Associate Attorney General of the United States, any Assistant Attorney General of the United States, or any employee of the Department of Justice or any employee of any department or agency of the United States so designated by the Attorney General to carry out the powers conferred on the Attorney General by this chapter. Any department or agency so designated may use in investigations authorized by this chapter either the investigative provisions of this chapter or the investigative power of such department or agency otherwise conferred by law.

E

Sample Child Abuse Reporting Laws

WI ST 48.981
West's Wisconsin Statutes Annotated
Social Services
Chapter 48. Children's Code
Subchapter XX. Miscellaneous Provisions

48.981 ABUSED OR NEGLECTED CHILDREN

Definitions. In This Section:

"Caregiver" means, with respect to a child who is the victim or alleged victim of abuse or neglect or who is threatened with abuse or neglect, any of the following persons:

(1) The child's parent, grandparent, stepparent, brother, sister, stepbrother, stepsister, half brother or half sister.

(2) The child's guardian.

(3) The child's legal custodian.

(4) A person who resides or has resided regularly or intermittently in the same dwelling as the child.

(5) An employee of a residential facility or child caring institution in which the child was or is placed.

(6) A person who provides or has provided care for the child in or outside of the child's home.

(7) Any other person who exercises or has exercised temporary or permanent control over the child or who temporarily or permanently supervises or has supervised the child.

(8) Any relative of the child other than a relative specified in subd. 1.

"Indian child" means any unmarried person who is under the age of 18 years and is affiliated with an Indian tribe or band in any of the following ways:

(1) As a member of the tribe or band.

(2) As a person who is both eligible for membership in the tribe or band and is the biological child of a member of the tribe or band.

(d) "Neglect" means failure, refusal or inability on the part of a parent, guardian, legal custodian or other person exercising temporary or permanent control over a child, for reasons other than poverty, to provide necessary care, food, clothing, medical or dental care or shelter so as to seriously endanger the physical health of the child.

(f) "Record" means any document relating to the investigation, assessment and disposition of a report under this section.

"Relative" means a parent, grandparent, stepparent, brother, sister, first cousin, 2nd cousin, nephew, niece, uncle, aunt, stepgrandparent, stepbrother, stepsister, half brother, half sister, brother in law, sister in law, stepuncle or stepaunt.

(g) "Reporter" means a person who reports suspected abuse or neglect or a belief that abuse or neglect will occur under this section.

(h) "Subject" means a person named in a report or record as either of the following:

(1) A child who is the victim or alleged victim of abuse or neglect or who is threatened with abuse or neglect.

(2) A person who is suspected of abuse or neglect or who has been determined to have abused or neglected a child.

(i) "Tribal agent" means the person designated under 25 CFR 23.12 by an Indian tribe or band to receive notice of involuntary child custody proceedings under the Indian child welfare act, 25 USC 1901 to 1963.

(2) Persons required to report. A physician, coroner, medical examiner, nurse, dentist, chiropractor, optometrist, acupuncturist, other medical or mental health professional, social worker, marriage and family therapist, professional counselor, public assistance worker, including a financial and employment planner, as defined in s. 49.141(1)(d), school teacher, administrator or counselor, mediator under s. 767.11, child care worker in a day care center or child caring institution, day care provider, alcohol or other drug abuse counselor, member of the treatment staff employed by or working under contract with a county department under s. 46.23, 51.42 or 51.437, physical therapist, occupational therapist, dietitian, speech-language pathologist, audiologist, emergency medical technician or police or law enforcement officer having reasonable cause to suspect that a child seen in the course of professional duties has been abused or neglected or having reason to believe that a child seen in the course of professional duties has been threatened with abuse or neglect and that abuse or neglect of the child will occur shall, except as provided under sub. (2m), report as provided in sub. (3). Any other person, including an attorney, having reason to suspect that a child has been abused or neglected or reason to believe that a child has been threatened with abuse or neglect and that abuse or neglect of the child will occur may make such a report. No person making a report under this subsection may be discharged from employment for so doing.

Exception to reporting requirement. (a) The purpose of this subsection is to allow children to obtain confidential health care services.

(b) In this subsection:

(1) "Health care provider" means a physician, as defined under s. 448.01(5), a physician assistant, as defined under s. 448.01(6), or a nurse holding a certificate of registration under s. 441.06(1) or a license under s. 441.10(3).

(2) "Health care service" means family planning services, pregnancy testing, obstetrical health care or screening, diagnosis and treatment for a sexually transmitted disease.

(c) Except as provided under pars. (d) and (e), the following persons are not required to report as suspected or threatened abuse, as defined in s. 48.02(1)(b), sexual intercourse or sexual contact involving a child:

(1) A health care provider who provides any health care service to a child.

(2) A person who obtains information about a child who is receiving or has received health care services from a health care provider.

(d) Any person described under par. (c)1. or 4. shall report as required under sub. (2) if he or she has reason to suspect any of the following:

(1) That the sexual intercourse or sexual contact occurred or is likely to occur with a caregiver.

(2) That the child suffered or suffers from a mental illness or mental deficiency that rendered or renders the child temporarily or permanently incapable of understanding or evaluating the consequences of his or her actions.

(3) That the child, because of his or her age or immaturity, was or is incapable of understanding the nature or consequences of sexual intercourse or sexual contact.

(4) That the child was unconscious at the time of the act or for any other reason was physically unable to communicate unwillingness to engage in sexual intercourse or sexual contact.

(5) That another participant in the sexual contact or sexual intercourse was or is exploiting the child.

(e) In addition to the reporting requirements under par. (d), a person described under par. (c)1. or 4. shall report as required under sub. (2) if he or she has any reasonable doubt as to the voluntariness of the child's participation in the sexual contact or sexual intercourse.

(3) Reports; investigation. (a) Referral of report. A person required to report under sub. (2) shall immediately inform, by telephone or personally, the

county department or the sheriff or city, village or town police department of the facts and circumstances contributing to a suspicion of child abuse or neglect or to a belief that abuse or neglect will occur. The sheriff or police department shall within 12 hours, exclusive of Saturdays, Sundays or legal holidays, refer to the county department all cases reported to it. The county department may require that a subsequent report be made in writing. Each county department shall adopt a written policy specifying the kinds of reports it will routinely report to local law enforcement authorities.

(b) Duties of local law enforcement agencies.

(1) Any person reporting under this section may request an immediate investigation by the sheriff or police department if the person has reason to suspect that a child's health or safety is in immediate danger. Upon receiving such a request, the sheriff or police department shall immediately investigate to determine if there is reason to believe that the child's health or safety is in immediate danger and take any necessary action to protect the child.

(2) If the investigating officer has reason under s. 48.19(1)(c) or (d)5. to take a child into custody, the investigating officer shall take the child into custody and deliver the child to the intake worker under s. 48.20.

(3) If the police or other law enforcement officials determine that criminal action is necessary, they shall refer the case to the district attorney for criminal prosecution.

APPENDIX

F

CHAMPUS Authorized Provider Definition Form and Federal Regulations

32 CFR § 199.2
Code of Federal Regulations
Title 32 National Defense
Subtitle A Department of Defense
Chapter I Office of the Secretary of Defense
Subchapter Miscellaneous
Part 199 Civilian Health and Medical Program of the Uniformed Services (CHAMPUS)
63 FR 17812

§ 199.2 DEFINITIONS

(a) General. In an effort to be as specific as possible as to the word and intent of CHAMPUS, the following definitions have been developed. While many of the definitions are general and some assign meaning to relatively common terms within the health insurance environment, others are applicable only to CHAMPUS; however, they all appear in this part solely for the purpose of the Program. Except when otherwise specified, the definitions in this section apply generally throughout this part.

Occupational therapist. A person who is trained specially in the skills and techniques of occupational therapy (that is, the use of purposeful activity with individuals who are limited by physical injury of illness, psychosocial dysfunction, developmental or learning disabilities, poverty and cultural differ-

ences, or the aging process in order to maximize independence, prevent disability, and maintain health) and who is licensed to administer occupational therapy treatments prescribed by a physician.

32 CFR § 199.6
Code of Federal Regulations
Title 32 National Defense
Subtitle A Department of Defense
Chapter I Office of the Secretary of Defense
Subchapter Miscellaneous
Part 199 Civilian Health and Medical Program of the Uniformed Services (CHAMPUS)

§ 199.6 AUTHORIZED PROVIDERS

(a) General. This section sets forth general policies and procedures that are the basis for the CHAMPUS costsharing of medical services and supplies provided by institutions, individuals, or other types of providers. Providers seeking payment from the Federal Government through programs such as CHAMPUS have a duty to familiarize themselves with, and comply with, the program requirements.

(1) Licensed registered nurses.
(c) (3) (iii) (I) (2)
(2) Licensed practical or vocational nurses.
(c) (3) (iii) (I) (3)

(3) Licensed registered physical therapists and occupational therapists.

(c) (3) (iii) (I) (4)

(4) Audiologists.

(c) (3) (iii) (I) (5)

(5) Speech therapists (speech pathologists).

(c) (3) (iv)

Authors' comment: This regulation does not include assistants as "authorized providers."

G

Medicare Regulation's Definition of Skilled Care in Home Care

42 CFR § 409.44

Code of Federal Regulations
Title 42 Public Health
Chapter IV Health Care Financing Administration, Department of Health and Human Services
    Subchapter B Medicare Program
    Part 409 Hospital Insurance Benefits
    Subpart E Home Health Services Under Hospital Insurance
    Excerpts:

§ 409.44 SKILLED SERVICES REQUIREMENTS

(a) General. The intermediary's decision on whether care is reasonable and necessary is based on information provided on the forms and in the medical record concerning the unique medical condition of the individual beneficiary. A coverage denial is not made solely on the basis of the reviewer's general inferences about patients with similar diagnoses or on data related to utilization generally but is based upon objective clinical evidence regarding the beneficiary's individual need for care.

Authors' comment: (b), omitted from this excerpt, pertains to skilled nursing care.

(c) Physical therapy, speech-language pathology services, and occupational therapy. To be covered, physical therapy, speech-language pathology services, and occupational therapy must satisfy the criteria in paragraphs (c)(1) through (4) of this section. Occupational therapy services initially qualify for home health coverage only if they are part of a plan of care that also includes intermittent skilled nursing care, physical therapy, or speech language pathology services as follows:

(1) Speech-language pathology services and physical or occupational therapy services must relate directly and specifically to a treatment regimen (established by the physician, after any needed consultation with the qualified therapist) that is designed to treat the beneficiary's illness or injury. Services related to activities for the general physical welfare of beneficiaries (for example, exercises to promote overall fitness) do not constitute physical therapy, occupational therapy, or speech-language pathology services for Medicare purposes.

(2) Physical and occupational therapy and speech-language pathology services must be reasonable and necessary. To be considered reasonable and necessary, the following conditions must be met:

    (i) The services must be considered under accepted standards of medical practice to be a specific, safe, and effective treatment for the beneficiary's condition.

(ii) The services must be of such a level of complexity and sophistication or the condition of the beneficiary must be such that the services required can safely and effectively be performed only by a qualified physical therapist or by a qualified physical therapy assistant under the supervision of a qualified physical therapist, by a qualified speech-language pathologist, or by a qualified occupational therapist or a qualified occupational therapy assistant under the supervision of a qualified occupational therapist (as defined in § 484.4 of this chapter). Services that do not require the performance or supervision of a physical therapist or an occupational therapist are not considered reasonable or necessary physical therapy or occupational therapy services, even if they are performed by or supervised by a physical therapist or occupational therapist. Services that do not require the skills of a speech-language pathologist are not considered to be reasonable and necessary speech-language pathology services even if they are performed by or supervised by a speech-language pathologist.

(iii) There must be an expectation that the beneficiary's condition will improve materially in a reasonable (and generally predictable) period of time based on the physician's assessment of the beneficiary's restoration potential and unique medical condition, or the services must be necessary to establish a safe and effective maintenance program required in connection with a specific disease, or the skills of a therapist must be necessary to perform a safe and effective maintenance program. If the services are for the establishment of a maintenance program, they may include the design of the program, the instruction of the beneficiary, family, or home health aides, and the necessary infrequent reevaluations of the beneficiary and the program to the degree that the specialized knowledge and judgment of a physical therapist, speech-language pathologist, or occupational therapist is required.

(iv) The amount, frequency, and duration of the services must be reasonable.

H

Medicare Regulation's Definition of Skilled Services in Post-Hospital SNFs

42 CFR § 409.33

Code of Federal Regulations
Title 42 Public Health
Chapter IV Health Care Financing Administration, Department of Health and Human Services
Subchapter B Medicare Program
Part 409 Hospital Insurance Benefits
Subpart D Requirements For Coverage of Post-hospital SNF Care

§ 409.33 Examples of Skilled Nursing and Rehabilitation Services

(a) Services that could qualify as either skilled nursing or skilled rehabilitation services:

(1) Overall management and evaluation of care plan. The development, management, and evaluation of a patient care plan based on the physician's orders constitute skilled services when, because of the patient's physical or mental condition, those activities require the involvement of technical or professional personnel in order to meet the patient's needs, promote recovery, and ensure medical safety. This would included the management of a plan involving only a variety of personal care services when, in light of the patient's condition, the aggregate of those ser-

vices requires the involvement of technical or professional personnel. For example, an aged patient with a history of diabetes mellitus and angina pectoris who is recovering from an open reduction of a fracture of the neck of the femur requires, among other services, careful skin care, appropriate oral medications, a diabetic diet, an exercise program to preserve muscle tone and body condition, and observation to detect signs of deterioration in his or her condition or complications resulting from restricted, but increasing, mobility. Although any of the required services could be performed by a properly instructed person, such a person would not have the ability to understand the relationship between the services and evaluate the ultimate effect of one service on the other. Since the nature of the patient's condition, age, and immobility create a high potential for serious complications, such an understanding is essential to ensure the patient's recovery and safety. Under these circumstances, the management of the plan of care would require the skills of a nurse even though the individual services are not skilled. Skilled planning and management activities are not always specifically identified in the patient's clinical record. Therefore, if the patient's overall condition would support a finding that recovery and safety can be assured only if the total care is planned, managed, and evaluated by technical or professional personnel, it would be appropriate to infer that skilled services are being provided.

(2) Observation and assessment of the patient's changing condition. Observation and assessment constitute skilled services when the skills of a technical or professional person are required to identify and evaluate the patient's need for modification of treatment for additional medical procedures until his or her condition is stabilized. For example, a patient with congestive heart failure may require continuous close observation to detect signs of decompensation, abnormal fluid balance, or adverse effects resulting from prescribed medication(s) which serve as indicators for adjusting therapeutic measures. Likewise, surgical patients transferred from a hospital to a skilled nursing facility while in the complicated, unstabilized postoperative period, e.g., after hip prosthesis or cataract surgery, may need continued close skilled monitoring for postoperative complications, and adverse reaction. Patients who, in addition to their physical problems, exhibit acute psychological symptoms such as depression, anxiety, or agitation, etc., may also require skilled observation and assessment by technical or professional personnel to assure their safety and/or the safety of others, i.e., to observe for indications of suicidal or hostile behavior. The need for services of this type must be documented by physicians' orders and/or nursing or therapy notes.

(3) Patient education services. Patient education services are skilled services if the use of technical or professional personnel is necessary to teach a patient self-maintenance. For example, a patient who has had a recent leg amputation needs skilled rehabilitation services provided by technical or professional personnel to provide gait training and to teach prosthesis care. Likewise, a patient newly diagnosed with diabetes requires instruction from technical or professional personnel to learn the self-administration of insulin or footcare precautions, etc.

Authors' comment: (b) is omitted from this excerpt; it pertains to nursing care.

(c) Services which would qualify as skilled rehabilitation services.

(1) Ongoing assessment of rehabilitation needs and potential: Services concurrent with the management of a patient care plan, including tests and measurements of range of motion, strength, balance, coordination, endurance, functional ability, activities of daily living, perceptual deficits, speech and language or hearing disorders;

(2) Therapeutic exercises or activities: Therapeutic exercises or activities which, because of the type of exercises employed or the condition of the patient, must be performed by or under the supervision of a qualified physical therapist or occupational therapist to ensure the safety of the patient and the effectiveness of the treatment;

(3) Gait evaluation and training: Gait evaluation and training furnished to restore function in a patient whose ability to walk has been impaired by neurological, muscular, or skeletal abnormality;

(4) Range of motion exercises: Range of motion exercises which are part of the active treatment of a specific disease state which has resulted in a loss of, or restriction of, mobility (as evidenced by a therapist's notes showing the degree of motion lost and the degree to be restored);

(5) Maintenance therapy; Maintenance therapy, when the specialized knowledge and judgment of a qualified therapist is required to design and establish a maintenance program based on an initial evaluation and periodic reassessment of the patient's needs, and consistent with the patient's capacity and tolerance. For example, a patient with Parkinson's disease who has not been under a rehabilitation regimen may require the services of a qualified therapist to determine what type of exercises will contribute the most to the maintenance of his present level of functioning.

(6) Ultrasound, shortwave, and microwave therapy treatment by a qualified physical therapist;

(7) Hot pack, hydrocollator, infrared treatments, paraffin baths, and whirlpool; Hot pack hydrocollator, infrared treatments, paraffin baths, and whirlpool in particular cases where the patient's condition is complicated by circulatory deficiency, areas of desensitization, open wounds, fractures, or other complications, and the skills, knowledge, and judgment of a qualified physical therapist are required; and

(8) Services of a speech pathologist or audiologist when necessary for the restoration of function in speech or hearing.

(d) Personal care services. Personal care services which do not require the skills of qualified technical or professional personnel are not skilled services except under the circumstances specified in § 409.32

(b). Personal care services include, but are not limited to, the following:

(1) Administration of routine oral medications, eye drops, and ointments;

(2) General maintenance care of colostomy and ileostomy;

(3) Routine services to maintain satisfactory functioning of indwelling bladder catheters;

(4) Changes of dressing for noninfected postoperative or chronic conditions;

(5) Prophylactic and palliative skin care, including bathing and application of creams, or treatment of minor skin problems;

(6) Routine care of the incontinent patient, including use of diapers and protective sheets;

(7) General maintenance care in connection with a plaster cast;

(8) Routine care in connection with braces and similar devices;

(9) Use of heat as a palliative and comfort measure, such as whirlpool and hydrocollator;

(10) Routine administration of medical gases after a regimen of therapy has been established;

(11) Assistance in dressing, eating, and going to the toilet;

(12) Periodic turning and positioning in bed; and

(13) General supervision of exercises which have been taught to the patient; including the actual carrying out of maintenance programs, i.e., the performance of the repetitive exercises required to maintain function do not require the skills of a therapist and would not constitute skilled rehabilitation services (see paragraph (c) of this section). Similarly, repetitious exercises to improve gait, maintain strength, or endurance; passive exercises to maintain range of motion in paralyzed extremities, which are not related to a specific loss of function; and assistive walking do not constitute skilled rehabilitation services.

Criminal Penalties for Fraud Against a Federal Health Care Program

42 USCA § 1320A-7B

United States Code Annotated
Title 42 The Public Health and Welfare
Chapter 7 Social Security
Subchapter XI General Provisions, Peer Review, and Administrative Simplification
Part A General Provisions

§ 1320a-7b Criminal Penalties for Acts Involving Federal Health Care Programs

(a) Making or causing to be made false statements or representations

Whoever—

(1) knowingly and willfully makes or causes to be made any false statement or representation of a material fact in any application for any benefit or payment under a Federal health care program (as defined in subsection (f) of this section),

(2) at any time knowingly and willfully makes or causes to be made any false statement or representation of a material fact for use in determining rights to such benefit or payment,

(3) having knowledge of the occurrence of any event affecting (A) his initial or continued right to any such benefit or payment, or (B) the initial or continued right to any such benefit or payment of any other individual in whose behalf he has applied for or is receiving such benefit or payment, conceals or fails to disclose such event with an intent fraudulently to secure such benefit or payment either in a greater amount or quantity than is due or when no such benefit or payment is authorized,

(4) having made application to receive any such benefit or payment for the use and benefit of another and having received it, knowingly and willfully converts such benefit or payment or any part thereof to a use other than for the use and benefit of such other person,

(5) presents or causes to be presented a claim for a physician's service for which payment may be made under a Federal health care program and knows that the individual who furnished the service was not licensed as a physician, or

(6) for a fee knowingly and willfully counsels or assists an individual to dispose of assets (including by any transfer in trust) in order for the individual to become eligible for medical assistance under a State plan under subchapter XIX of this chapter, if disposing of the assets results in the imposition of a period of ineligibility for such assistance under section 1396p(c) of this title,

shall (i) in the case of such a statement, representation, concealment, failure, or conversion by any person in connection with the furnishing (by that person) of items or services for which payment is or may be made under the program, be guilty of a felony and upon conviction thereof fined not more than $25,000 or imprisoned for not more than five years or both, or (ii) in the case of such a statement, representation, concealment, failure, conversion, or provision of counsel or assistance by any other person, be guilty of a misdemeanor and upon conviction thereof fined not more than $10,000 or imprisoned for not more than one year, or both. In addition, in any case where an individual who is otherwise eligible for assistance under a Federal health care program is convicted of an offense under the preceding provisions of this subsection, the administrator of such program may at its option (notwithstanding any other provision of such program) limit, restrict, or suspend the eligibility of that individual for such period (not exceeding one year) as it deems appropriate; but the imposition of a limitation, restriction, or suspension with respect to the eligibility of any individual under this sentence shall not affect the eligibility of any other person for assistance under the plan, regardless of the relationship between that individual and such other person.

(b) Illegal remunerations

(1) whoever knowingly and willfully solicits or receives any remuneration (including any kickback, bribe, or rebate) directly or indirectly, overtly or covertly, in cash or in kind-

(A) in return for referring an individual to a person for the furnishing or arranging for the furnishing of any item or service for which payment may be made in whole or in part under a Federal health care program, or

(B) in return for purchasing, leasing, ordering, or arranging for or recommending purchasing, leasing, or ordering any good, facility, service, or item for which payment may be made in whole or in part under a Federal health care program,

shall be guilty of a felony and upon conviction thereof, shall be fined not more than $25,000 or imprisoned for not more than five years, or both.

(2) whoever knowingly and willfully offers or pays any remuneration (including any kickback, bribe, or rebate) directly or indirectly, overtly or covertly, in cash or in kind to any person to induce such person—

(A) to refer an individual to a person for the furnishing or arranging for the furnishing of any item or service for which payment may be made in whole or in part under a Federal health care program, or

(B) to purchase, lease, order, or arrange for or recommend purchasing, leasing, or ordering any good, facility, service, or item for which payment may be made in whole or in part under a Federal health care program,

shall be guilty of a felony and upon conviction thereof, shall be fined not more than $25,000 or imprisoned for not more than five years, or both.

(3) Paragraphs (1) and (2) shall not apply to-

(A) a discount or other reduction in price obtained by a provider of services or other entity under a Federal health care program if the reduction in price is properly disclosed and appropriately reflected in the costs claimed or charges made by the provider or entity under a Federal health care program;

(B) any amount paid by an employer to an employee (who has a bona fide employment relationship with such employer) for employment in the provision of covered items or services;

(C) any amount paid by a vendor of goods or services to a person authorized to act as a purchasing agent for a group of individuals or entities who are furnishing services reimbursed under a Federal health care program if—

(i) the person has a written contract, with each such individual or entity, which specifies the amount to be paid the person, which amount may be a fixed amount or a fixed percentage of the value of the purchases made by each such individual or entity under the contract, and

(ii) in the case of an entity that is a provider of services (as defined in section 1395x(u) of this title), the person discloses (in such form and manner as the Secretary requires) to the entity and, upon request, to the Secretary the amount received from each such vendor with respect to purchases made by or on behalf of the entity;

(D) a waiver of any coinsurance under part B of subchapter XVIII of this chapter by a Federally qualified health care center with respect to an individual who qualifies for subsidized services under a provision of the Public Health Service Act [42 USCA § 201 et seq.];

(E) any payment practice specified by the Secretary in regulations promulgated pursuant to section 14(a) of the Medicare and Medicaid Patient and Program Protection Act of 1987; and

(F) any remuneration between an organization and an individual or entity providing items or services, or a combination thereof, pursuant to a written agreement between the organization and the individual or entity if the organization is an eligible organization under section 1395mm of this title or if the written agreement, through a risk-sharing arrangement, places the individual or entity at substantial financial risk for the cost or utilization of the items or services, or a combination thereof, which the individual or entity is obligated to provide.

(c) False statements or representations with respect to condition or operation of institutions

Whoever knowingly and willfully makes or causes to be made, or induces or seeks to induce the making of, any false statement or representation of a material fact with respect to the conditions or operation of any institution, facility, or entity in order that such institution, facility, or entity may qualify (either upon initial certification or upon recertification) as a hospital, critical access hospital, skilled nursing facility, nursing facility, intermediate care facility for the mentally retarded, home health agency, or other entity (including an eligible organization under section 1395mm(b) of this title) for which certification is required under subchapter XVIII of this chapter or a State health care program (as defined in section 1320a-7(h) of this title), or with respect to information required to be provided under section 1320a-3a of this title, shall be guilty of a felony and upon conviction thereof shall be fined not more than $25,000 or imprisoned for not more than five years, or both.

(d) Illegal patient admittance and retention practices

Whoever knowingly and willfully—

(1) charges, for any service provided to a patient under a State plan approved under subchapter XIX of this chapter, money or other consideration at a rate

in excess of the rates established by the State (or, in the case of services provided to an individual enrolled with a Medicaid managed care organization under subchapter XIX of this chapter under a contract under section 1396b(m) of this title or under a contractual, referral, or other arrangement under such contract, at a rate in excess of the rate permitted under such contract), or

(2) charges, solicits, accepts, or receives, in addition to any amount otherwise required to be paid under a State plan approved under subchapter XIX of this chapter, any gift, money, donation, or other consideration (other than a charitable, religious, or philanthropic contribution from an organization or from a person unrelated to the patient)-

(A) as a precondition of admitting a patient to a hospital, nursing facility, or intermediate care facility for the mentally retarded, or

(B) as a requirement for the patient's continued stay in such a facility,

when the cost of the services provided therein to the patient is paid for (in whole or in part) under the State plan,

shall be guilty of a felony and upon conviction thereof shall be fined not more than $25,000 or imprisoned for not more than five years, or both.

(e) Violation of assignment terms

Whoever accepts assignments described in section 1395u(b)(3)(B)(ii) of this title or agrees to be a participating physician or supplier under section 1395u(h)(1) of this title and knowingly, willfully, and repeatedly violates the term of such assignments or agreement, shall be guilty of a misdemeanor and upon conviction thereof shall be fined not more than $2,000 or imprisoned for not more than six months, or both.

(f) "Federal health care program" defined

For purposes of this section, the term "Federal health care program" means-

(1) any plan or program that provides health benefits, whether directly, through insurance, or otherwise, which is funded directly, in whole or in part, by the United States Government (other than the health insurance program under chapter 89 of Title 5); or

(2) any State health care program, as defined in section 1320a-7(h) of this title.

J

Sexual Harassment Information

THREE ELEMENTS OF SEXUAL HARASSMENT

1. Unwanted or unwelcome behavior.
2. Behavior is sexual or gender related.
3. Behavior occurs in a relationship where one person has more formal or informal power over the other.

FOUR CONDITIONS THAT GIVE RISE TO SEXUAL HARASSMENT

1. Submission to the conduct is made a term or condition, either explicitly or implicitly, of obtaining employment; or
2. Submission or rejection of the conduct is used as a factor in decisions affecting that person's employment; or
3. The conduct has either the purpose or effect of "substantially interfering" with a person's employment; or
4. The conduct creates an "intimidating, hostile, or offensive" work environment.

K

Independent Contractor Tests and IRS Revenue Ruling

COMMON LAW FACTORS FOR INDEPENDENT CONTRACTOR TEST

1. The extent of control the "employer" may exercise over the details of the work under the agreement
2. Whether or not the employee is engaged in a district occupation
3. The kind of occupation and whether the work is usually performed under the supervision of the employer or by a specialist without supervision
4. The amount and extent the particular occupation requires skill
5. Whether the employer supplies the tools and place of work for the worker
6. The length of time the worker is employed
7. Whether the employer pays the worker by time or by the job
8. Whether the work is part of the regular business of the employer
9. Whether the parties believe by their actions they are creating an employment relationship
10. Whether or not the principal is in business

EMPLOYEE-INDEPENDENT CONTRACTOR TEST: 20 FACTORS USED BY THE IRS

1. Compliance with employer instructions
2. Training provided by employer to perform job in a particular manner
3. Integration of services into business operations
4. Services personally rendered by the contractor/worker
5. Hiring, supervising and paying assistants
6. Continuing relationship between worker and the person for whom services are provided
7. Set work hours
8. Full-time hours required
9. Work performed on employer's premises
10. Services performed in a set order of sequence
11. Required written or oral reports
12. Payment by the hour, week, or job
13. Reimbursement for business or travel expenses
14. Furnishing of tools and materials
15. Significant investment in the facilities used to perform services

16. Realization of profits or losses
17. Working for more than one firm at a time
18. Making services available to the general public
19. Right to discharge for reasons other than nonperformance to contract specifications
20. Right to terminate relationship without incurring liability for failure to complete the job

EMPLOYMENT STATUS UNDER SECTION 530(D) OF THE REVENUE ACT OF 1978

Rev. Rul. 8741
1987-1 C.B. 296, 1987 WL 419174 (IRS)
Internal Revenue Service (IRS) Revenue Ruling
Published: 1987

Section 3121 Definitions, 26 CFR 31.3121(d)1: Who are Employees?

(Also Sections 3306, 3401; 31.3306(i)1, 31.3401(c)1.)

Employment status under section 530(d) of the Revenue Act of 1978. Guidelines are set forth for determining the employment status of a taxpayer (technical service specialist) affected by section 530(d) of the Revenue Act of 1978, as added by section 1706 of the Tax Reform Act of 1986. The specialists are to be classified as employees under generally applicable common law standards.

Issue

In the situations described below, are the individuals employees under the common law rules for purposes of the Federal Insurance Contributions Act (FICA), the Federal Unemployment Tax Act (FUTA), and the Collection of Income Tax at Source on Wages (chapters 21, 23, and 24 respectively, subtitle C, Internal Revenue Code)? These situations illustrate the application of section 530(d) of the Revenue Act of 1978, 19783 (Vol. 1) C.B. xi, 119 (the 1978 Act), which was added by section 1706(a) of the Tax Reform Act of 1986, 19863 (Vol. 1) C.B. (the 1986 Act) (generally effective for services performed and remuneration paid after December 31, 1986).

Facts

In each factual situation, an individual worker (Individual), pursuant to an arrangement between one person (Firm) and another person (Client), provides services for the Client as an engineer, designer, drafter, computer programmer, systems analyst, or other similarly skilled worker engaged in a similar line of work.

Situation 1

The Firm is engaged in the business of providing temporary technical services to its clients. The Firm maintains a roster of workers who are available to provide technical services to prospective clients. The Firm does not train the workers but determines the services that the workers are qualified to perform based on information submitted by the workers.

The Firm has entered into a contract with the Client. The contract states that the Firm is to provide the Client with workers to perform computer programming services meeting specified qualifications for a particular project. The Individual, a computer programmer, enters into a contract with the Firm to perform services as a computer programmer for the Client's project, which is expected to last less than one year. The Individual is one of several programmers provided by the Firm to the Client. The Individual has not been an employee of or performed services for the Client (or any predecessor or affiliated corporation of the Client) at any time preceding the time at which the Individual begins performing services for the Client. Also, the Individual has not been an employee of or performed services for or on behalf of the Firm at any time preceding the time at which the Individual begins performing services for the Client. The Individual's contract with the Firm states that the Individual is an independent contractor with respect to services performed on behalf of the Firm for the Client.

The Individual and the other programmers perform the services under the Firm's contract with the Client. During the time the Individual is performing services for the Client, even though the Individual retains the right to perform services for other persons, substantially all of the Individual's working time is devoted to performing services for the Client. A significant portion of the services are performed on the Client's premises. The Individual reports to the Firm by accounting for time worked and describing the progress of the work. The Firm pays the Individual and regularly charges the Client for the services performed by the Individual. The Firm generally does not pay individuals who perform services for the Client unless the Firm provided such individuals to the Client.

The work of the Individual and other programmers is regularly reviewed by the Firm. The review is based primarily on reports by the Client about the performance of these workers. Under the contract between the Individual and the Firm, the Firm may terminate its relationship with the Individual if the review shows that he or she is failing to perform the services contracted for by the Client. Also, the Firm will replace the Individual with another worker if the Individual's services are unacceptable to the Client. In such a case, however, the Individual will nevertheless receive his or her hourly pay for the work completed.

Finally, under the contract between the Individual and the Firm, the Individual is prohibited from performing services directly for the Client and, under the contract between the Firm and the Client, the Client is prohibited from receiving services from the Individual for a period of three months following the termination or services by the Individual for the Client on behalf of the Firm.

Situation 2

The Firm is a technical services firm that supplies clients with technical personnel. The Client requires the services of a systems analyst to complete a project and contacts the Firm to obtain such an analyst. The Firm maintains a roster of analysts and refers such an analyst, the Individual, to the Client. The Individual is not restricted by the Client or the Firm from providing services to the general public while performing services for the Client and in fact does perform substantial services for other persons during the period the Individual is working for the Client. Neither the Firm nor the Client has priority on the services of the Individual. The Individual does not report, directly or indirectly, to the Firm after the beginning of the assignment to the Client concerning (1) hours worked by the Individual, (2) progress on the job, or (3) expenses incurred by the Individual in performing services for the Client. No reports (including reports of time

worked or progress on the job) made by the Individual to the Client are provided by the Client to the Firm.

If the Individual ceases providing services for the Client prior to completion of the project or if the Individual's work product is otherwise unsatisfactory, the Client may seek damages from the Individual. However, in such circumstances, the Client may not seek damages from the Firm, and the Firm is not required to replace the Individual. The Firm may not terminate the services of the Individual while he or she is performing services for the Client and may not otherwise affect the relationship between the Client and the Individual. Neither the Individual nor the Client is prohibited for any period after termination of the Individual's services on this job from contracting directly with the other. For referring the Individual to the Client, the Firm receives a flat fee that is fixed prior to the Individual's commencement of services for the Client and is unrelated to the number of hours and quality of work performed by the Individual. The Individual is not paid by the Firm either directly or indirectly. No payment made by the Client to the Individual reduces the amount of the fee that the Client is otherwise required to pay the Firm. The Individual is performing services that can be accomplished without the Individual's receiving direction or control as to hours, place of work, sequence, or details of work.

Situation 3

The Firm, a company engaged in furnishing client firms with technical personnel, is contacted by the Client, who is in need of the services of a drafter for a particular project, which is expected to last less than one year. The Firm recruits the Individual to perform the drafting services for the Client. The Individual performs substantially all of the services for the Client at the office of the Client, using materials and equipment of the Client. The services are performed under the supervision of employees of the Client. The Individual reports to the Client on a regular basis. The Individual is paid by the Firm based on the number of hours the Individual has worked for the Client, as reported to the Firm by the Client or as reported by the Individual and confirmed by the Client. The Firm has no obligation to pay the Individual if the Firm does not receive payment for the Individual's services from the Client. For recruiting the Individual for the Client, the Firm receives a flat fee that is fixed prior to the Individual's commencement of services for the Client and is unrelated to the number of hours and quality of work performed by the Individual. However, the Firm does receive a reasonable fee for performing the payroll function. The Firm may not direct the work of the Individual and has no responsibility for the work performed by the Individual. The Firm may not terminate the services of the Individual. The Client may terminate the services of the Individual without liability to either the Individual or the Firm. The Individual is permitted to work for another firm while performing services for the Client, but does in fact work for the Client on a substantially full-time basis.

LAW AND ANALYSIS

This ruling provides guidance concerning the factors that are used to determine whether an employment relationship exists between the Individual and the Firm for federal employment tax purposes and applies those factors to the given factual situations to determine whether the Individual is an employee of the Firm for such purposes. The ruling does not reach any conclusions concerning whether an employment relationship for federal employment tax purposes exists between the Individual and the Client in any of the factual situations.

Analysis of the preceding three fact situations requires an examination of the common law rules for determining whether the Individual is an employee with respect to either the Firm or the Client, a determination of whether the Firm or the Client qualifies for employment tax relief under section 530(a) of the 1978 Act, and a determination of whether any such relief is denied the Firm under section 530(d) of the 1978 Act (added by Section 1706 of the 1986 Act).

An individual is an employee for federal employment tax purposes if the individual has the status of an employee under the usual common law rules applicable in determining the employer-employee relationship. Guides for determining that status are found in the following three substantially similar sections of the Employment Tax Regulations: sections 31.3121(d)1(c); 31.3306(i)1; and 31.3401(c)1.

These sections provide that generally the relationship of employer and employee exists when the person or persons for whom the services are performed have the right to control and direct the individual who performs the services, not only as to the result to be accomplished by the work but also as to the details and means by which that result is accomplished. That is, an employee is subject to the will and control of the employer not only as to what shall be done but as to how it shall be done. In this connection, it is not necessary that the employer actually direct or control the manner in which the services are performed; it is sufficient if the employer has the right to do so.

Conversely, these sections provide, in part, that individuals (such as physicians, lawyers, dentists, contractors, and subcontractors) who follow an independent trade, business, or profession, in which they offer their services to the public, generally are not employees.

Finally, if the relationship of employer and employee exists, the designation or description of the relationship by the parties as anything other than that of employer and employee is immaterial. Thus, if such a relationship exists, it is of no consequence that the employee is designated as a partner, coadventurer, agent, independent contractor, or the like.

As an aid to determining whether an individual is an employee under the common law rules, twenty factors or elements have been identified as indicating whether sufficient control is present to establish an employer-employee relationship. The twenty factors have been developed based on an examination of cases and rulings considering whether an individual is an employee. The degree of importance of each factor varies depending on the occupation and the factual context in which the services are performed. The twenty factors are designed only as guides for determining whether an individual is an employee; special scrutiny is required in applying the twenty factors to assure that formalistic aspects of an arrangement designed to achieve a particular status do not obscure the substance of the arrangement (that is, whether the person or persons for whom the services are performed exercise sufficient control over the individual for the individual to be classified as an employee). The twenty factors are described below:

(1) Instructions. A worker who is required to

comply with other persons' instructions about when, where, and how he or she is to work is ordinarily an employee. This control factor is present if the person or persons for whom the services are performed have the RIGHT to require compliance with instructions. See, for example, Rev. Rul. 68598, 19682 C.B. 464, and Rev. Rul. 66381, 19662 C.B. 449.

(2) Training. Training a worker by requiring an experienced employee to work with the worker, by corresponding with the worker, by requiring the worker to attend meetings, or by using other methods, indicates that the person or persons for whom the services are performed want the services performed in a particular method or manner. See Rev. Rul. 70630, 19702 C.B. 229.

(3) Integration. Integration of the worker's services into the business operations generally shows that the worker is subject to direction and control. When the success or continuation of a business depends to an appreciable degree upon the performance of certain services, the workers who perform those services must necessarily be subject to a certain amount of control by the owner of the business. See United States v. Silk, 331 U.S. 704 (1947), 19472 C.B. 167.

(4) Services rendered personally. If the Services must be rendered personally, presumably the person or persons for whom the services are performed are interested in the methods used to accomplish the work as well as in the results. See Rev. Rul. 55695, 19552 C.B. 410.

(5) Hiring, supervising, and paying assistants. If the person or persons for whom the services are performed hire, supervise, and pay assistants, that factor generally shows control over the workers on the job. However, if one worker hires, supervises, and pays the other assistants pursuant to a contract under which the worker agrees to provide materials and labor and under which the worker is responsible only for the attainment of a result, this factor indicates an independent contractor status. Compare Rev. Rul. 63115, 19631 C.B. 178, with Rev. Rul. 55593 19552 C.B. 610.

(6) Continuing relationship. A continuing relationship between the worker and the person or persons for whom the services are performed indicates that an employer-employee relationship exists. A continuing relationship may exist where work is per-

formed at frequently recurring although irregular intervals. See United States v. Silk.

(7) Set hours of work. The establishment of set hours of work by the person or persons for whom the services are performed is a factor indicating control. See Rev. Rul. 73591, 19732 C.B. 337.

(8) Full time required. If the worker must devote substantially full time to the business of the person or persons for whom the services are performed, such person or persons have control over the amount of time the worker spends working and impliedly restrict the worker from doing other gainful work. An independent contractor, on the other hand, is free to work when and for whom he or she chooses. See Rev. Rul. 56694, 19562 C.B. 694.

(9) Doing work on employer's premises. If the work is performed on the premises of the person or persons for whom the services are performed, that factor suggests control over the worker, especially if the work could be done elsewhere. Rev. Rul. 56660, 19562 C.B. 693. Work done off the premises of the person or persons receiving the services, such as at the office of the worker, indicates some freedom from control. However, this fact by itself does not mean that the worker is not an employee. The importance of this factor depends on the nature of the service involved and the extent to which an employer generally would require that employees perform such services on the employer's premises. Control over the place of work is indicated when the person or persons for whom the services are performed have the right to compel the worker to travel a designated route, to canvass a territory within a certain time, or to work at specific places as required. See Rev. Rul. 56694.

(10) Order or sequence set. If a worker must perform services in the order or sequence set by the person or persons for whom the services are performed, that factor shows that the worker is not free to follow the worker's own pattern of work but must follow the established routines and schedules of the person or persons for whom the services are performed. Often, because of the nature of an occupation, the person or persons for whom the services are performed do not set the order of the services or set the order infrequently. It is sufficient to show control, however, if such person or persons retain the right to do so. See Rev. Rul. 56694.

(11) Oral or written reports. A requirement that

the worker submit regular or written reports to the person or persons for whom the services are performed indicates a degree of control. See Rev. Rul. 70309, 19701 C.B. 199, and Rev. Rul. 68248, 19681 C.B. 431.

(12) Payment by hour, week, month. Payment by the hour, week, or month generally points to an employer-employee relationship, provided that this method of payment is not just a convenient way of paying a lump sum agreed upon as the cost of a job. Payment made by the job or on straight commission generally indicates that the worker is an independent contractor. See Rev. Rul. 74389, 19742 C.B. 330.

(13) Payment of business and/or traveling expenses. If the person or persons for whom the services are performed ordinarily pay the worker's business and/or traveling expenses, the worker is ordinarily an employee. An employer, to be able to control expenses, generally retains the right to regulate and direct the worker's business activities. See Rev. Rul. 55144, 19551 C.B. 483.

(14) Furnishing of tools and materials. The fact that the person or persons for whom the services are performed furnish significant tools, materials, and other equipment tends to show the existence of an employer-employee relationship. See Rev. Rul. 71524, 19712 C.B. 346.

(15) Significant investment. If the worker invests in facilities that are used by the worker in performing services and are not typically maintained by employees (such as the maintenance of an office rented at fair value from an unrelated party), that factor tends to indicate that the worker is an independent contractor. On the other hand, lack of investment in facilities indicates dependence on the person or persons for whom the services are performed for such facilities and, accordingly, the existence of an employer-employee relationship. See Rev. Rul. 71524. Special scrutiny is required with respect to certain types of facilities, such as home offices.

(16) Realization of profit or loss. A worker who can realize a profit or suffer a loss as a result of the worker's services (in addition to the profit or loss ordinarily realized by employees) is generally an independent contractor, but the worker who cannot is an employee. See Rev. Rul. 70309. For example, if the worker is subject to a real risk of economic loss due to significant investments or a bona fide liability for expenses, such as salary payments to unrelated employees, that factor indicates that the worker is an independent contractor. The risk that a worker will not receive payment for his or her services, however, is common to both independent contractors and employees and thus does not constitute a sufficient economic risk to support treatment as an independent contractor.

(17) Working for more than one firm at a time. If a worker performs more than de minimis services for a multiple of unrelated persons or firms at the same time, that factor generally indicates that the worker is an independent contractor. See Rev. Rul. 70572, 19702 C.B. 221. However, a worker who performs services for more than one person may be an employee of each of the persons, especially where such persons are part of the same service arrangement.

(18) Making service available to general public. The fact that a worker makes his or her services available to the general public on a regular and consistent basis indicates an independent contractor relationship. See Rev. Rul. 56660.

(19) Right to discharge. The right to discharge a worker is a factor indicating that the worker is an employee and the person possessing the right is an employer. An employer exercises control through the threat of dismissal, which causes the worker to obey the employer's instructions. An independent contractor, on the other hand, cannot be fired so long as the independent contractor produces a result that meets the contract specifications. Rev. Rul. 7541, 19751 C.B. 323.

(20) Right to terminate. If the worker has the right to end his or her relationship with the person for whom the services are performed at any time he or she wishes without incurring liability, that factor indicates an employer-employee relationship. See Rev. Rul. 70309.

Rev. Rul. 7541 considers the employment tax status of individuals performing services for a physician's professional service corporation. The corporation is in the business of providing a variety of services to professional people and firms (subscribers), including the services of secretaries, nurses, dental hygienists, and other similarly trained personnel. The individuals who are to perform the services are recruited by the corporation, paid by the corporation, assigned to jobs, and provided with employee benefits by the corporation. Individuals who enter into contracts with the corporation agree they will not contract directly with any subscriber to which they are assigned for at least three months after cessation of their contracts with the corporation. The corporation assigns the individual to the subscriber to work on the subscriber's premises with the subscriber's equipment. Subscribers have the right to require that an individual furnished by the corporation cease providing services to them, and they have the further right to have such individual replaced by the corporation within a reasonable period of time, but the subscribers have no right to affect the contract between the individual and the corporation. The corporation retains the right to discharge the individuals at any time. Rev. Rul. 7541 concludes that the individuals are employees of the corporation for federal employment tax purposes.

Rev. Rul. 70309 considers the employment tax status of certain individuals who perform services as oil well pumpers for a corporation under contracts that characterize such individuals as independent contractors. Even though the pumpers perform their services away from the headquarters of the corporation and are not given day-to-day directions and instructions, the ruling concludes that the pumpers are employees of the corporation because the pumpers perform their services pursuant to an arrangement that gives the corporation the right to exercise whatever control is necessary to assure proper performance of the services; the pumpers' services are both necessary and incident to the business conducted by the corporation; and the pumpers are not engaged in an independent enterprise in which they assume the usual business risks, but rather work in the course of the corporation's trade or business. See also Rev. Rul. 70630, 19702 C.B. 229, which considers the employment tax status of sales clerks furnished by an employee service company to a retail store to perform temporary services for the store.

Section 530(a) of the 1978 Act, as amended by section 269(c) of the Tax Equity and Fiscal Responsibility Act of 1982, 19822 C.B. 462, 536, provides, for purposes of the employment taxes under subtitle C of the Code, that if a taxpayer did not treat an individual as an employee for any period, then the individual shall be deemed not to be an employee, unless the taxpayer had no reasonable basis for not treating the individual as an employee.

For any period after December 31, 1978, this relief applies only if both of the following consistency rules are satisfied: (1) all federal tax returns (including information returns) required to be filed by the taxpayer with respect to the individual for the period are filed on a basis consistent with the taxpayer's treatment of the individual as not being an employee ("reporting consistency rule"), and (2) the taxpayer (and any predecessor) has not treated any individual holding a substantially similar position as an employee for purposes of the employment taxes for periods beginning after December 31, 1977 ("substantive consistency rule").

The determination of whether any individual who is treated as an employee holds a position substantially similar to the position held by an individual whom the taxpayer would otherwise be permitted to treat as other than an employee for employment tax purposes under section 530(a) of the 1978 Act requires an examination of all the facts and circumstances, including particularly the activities and functions performed by the individuals. Differences in the positions held by the respective individuals that result from the taxpayer's treatment of one individual as an employee and the other individual as other than an employee (for example, that the former individual is a participant in the taxpayer's qualified pension plan or health plan and the latter individual is not a participant in either) are to be disregarded in determining whether the individuals hold substantially similar positions.

Section 1706(a) of the 1986 Act added to section 530 of the 1978 Act a new subsection (d), which provides an exception with respect to the treatment of certain workers. Section 530(d) provides that section 530 shall not apply in the case of an individual who, pursuant to an arrangement between the taxpayer and another person, provides services for such other person as an engineer, designer, drafter, computer programmer, systems analyst, or other similarly skilled worker engaged in a similar line of work. Section 530(d) of the 1978 Act does not affect the determination of whether such workers are employees under the common law rules. Rather, it merely eliminates the employment tax relief under section 530(a) of the 1978 Act that would otherwise be available to a taxpayer with respect to those workers who are determined to be employees of the taxpayer under the usual common law rules. Section 530(d) applies to remuneration paid and services rendered after December 31, 1986.

The Conference Report on the 1986 Act discusses the effect of section 530(d) as follows:

The Senate amendment applies whether the services of [technical service workers] are provided by the firm to only one client during the year or to more than one client, and whether or not such individuals have been designated or treated by the technical services firm as independent contractors, sole proprietors, partners, or employees of a personal service corporation controlled by such individual. The effect of the provision cannot be avoided by claims that such technical service personnel are employees of personal service corporations controlled by such personnel. For example, an engineer retained by a technical services firm to provide services to a manufacturer cannot avoid the effect of this provision by organizing a corporation that he or she controls and then claiming to provide services as an employee of that corporation.

(The provision does not apply with respect to individuals who are classified, under the generally applicable common law standards, as employees of a business that is a client of the technical services firm; 2 H. R. Rep. No. 99841 [Conf. Rep.], 99th Cong., 2d Sess. II834 to 835 [1986].)

Under the facts of Situation 1 the legal relationship is between the Firm and the Individual, and the Firm retains the right of control to insure that the services are performed in a satisfactory fashion. The fact that the Client may also exercise some degree of control over the Individual does not indicate that the Individual is not an employee. Therefore, in Situation 1, the Individual is an employee of the Firm under the common law rules. The facts in Situation 1 involve an arrangement among the Individual, Firm, and Client, and the services provided by the Individual are technical services. Accordingly, the Firm is denied section 530 relief under section 530(d) of the 1978 Act (as added by section 1706 of the 1986 Act), and no relief is available with respect to any employment tax liability incurred in Situation 1. The analysis would not differ if the acts of Situation 1 were changed to state that the Individual provided the technical services through a personal service corporation owned by the Individual.

In Situation 2, the Firm does not retain any right to control the performance of the services by the Individual and, thus, no employment relationship exists between the Individual and the Firm.

In Situation 3, the Firm does not control the performance of the services of the Individual, and the Firm has no right to affect the relationship between the Client and the Individual. Consequently, no employment relationship exists between the Firm and the Individual.

HOLDINGS

Situation 1. The Individual is an employee of the Firm under the common law rules. Relief under section 530 of the 1978 Act is not available to the Firm because of the provisions of section 530(d).

Situation 2. The Individual is not an employee of the Firm under the common law rules.

Situation 3. The Individual is not an employee of the Firm under the common law rules.

Because of the application of section 530(b) of the 1978 Act, no inference should be drawn with respect to whether the Individual in Situations 2 and 3 is an employee of the Client for federal employment tax purposes (Rev. Rul. 8741).

L

Excerpt From the Health Insurance Manual for Home Health Agencies, HCFA, Fraud, and Abuse

07/92

106 FRAUD AND ABUSE— GENERAL

Providers and suppliers have an obligation, under law, to conform to the requirements of the Medicare program. Fraud and abuse committed against the program may be prosecuted under various provisions of the United States Code and could result in the imposition of restitution, fines, and, in some instances, imprisonment. In addition, there is also a range of administrative sanctions (such as exclusion from participation in the program) and civil monetary penalties that may be imposed when facts and circumstances warrant such action.

Following are definitions and examples of fraud and abuse. These definitions and examples give a better understanding of the types of practices that are forbidden, under law, in the Medicare program.

106.1 Definition and Examples of Fraud

Fraud is defined as making false statements or representations of material facts in order to obtain some benefit or payment for which no entitlement would otherwise exist. These acts may be committed either for the person's own benefit or for the benefit of some other party. In order to prove that fraud has been committed against the government, it is necessary to prove that fraudulent acts were performed knowingly, willfully, and intentionally.

Examples of fraud include, but are not limited to, the following:

- ◆ Billing for services that were not furnished and/or supplies not provided. This includes billing Medicare for appointments that the patient failed to keep;
- ◆ Altering claims forms and/or receipts in order to receive a higher payment amount;
- ◆ Duplicating billings that includes billing both the Medicare program and the beneficiary, Medicaid, or some other insurer in an effort to receive payment greater than allowed;
- ◆ Offering, paying, soliciting, or receiving bribes, kickbacks, or rebates, directly or indirectly, in cash or in kind, in order to induce referrals of patients or the purchase of goods or services that may be paid for by the Medicare program;
- ◆ Falsely representing the nature of the services furnished. This encompasses describing a noncovered service in a misleading way that makes it appear as if a covered service was actually furnished;
- ◆ Billing a person who has Medicare coverage for services provided to another person not eligible for Medicare coverage;

- Repeatedly violating the participation agreement, assignment agreement, and the maximum allowable actual charge (MAAC) limits or limitation amount;
- Completing certificates of medical necessity (CMN) for patients not personally and professionally known by the provider;
- Completing a prohibited CMN by suppliers;
- Using another person's Medicare card to obtain medical care;
- Giving false information about provider ownership in a clinical laboratory;
- Conspiring to submit or manipulate bills by a provider and a beneficiary, two or more providers and suppliers, or a provider and a carrier employee that results in higher costs or charges to the program;
- Billing procedures over a period of days when all treatment occurred during one visit (e.g., split billing schemes);
- Using the adjustment payment process to generate fraudulent payments; and
- Billing for "gang visits" (e.g., a physician visits a nursing home, walks through the facility, and bills for 20 nursing home visits without rendering any specific service to the individual patients).

106.2 Definition and Examples of Abuse

Abuse describes practices that, either directly or indirectly, result in unnecessary costs to the Medicare program. Many times abuse appears quite similar to fraud except that it is not possible to establish that abusive acts were committed knowingly, willfully, and intentionally.

Following are three standards that HCFA uses when judging whether abusive acts in billing were committed against the Medicare program:

- Medically necessary;
- Conform to professionally recognized standards; and
- Provided at a fair price.

Examples of abuse include, but are not limited to, the following:

- Charging in excess for services or supplies;
- Providing medically unnecessary services or services that do not meet professionally recognized standards;

- Billing Medicare based on a higher fee schedule than for non-Medicare patients;
- Submitting bills to Medicare that are the responsibility of other insurers under the Medicare secondary payer (MSP) regulation;
- Violating the participating physician/supplier agreement;
- Breaches in the assignment agreement; and
- Violating the MAAC or limitation amount.

Although these types of practices may initially be categorized as abusive in nature, under certain circumstances they may develop into fraud if there is evidence that the subject was knowingly and willfully conducting an abusive practice.

106.3 Responsibility for Combating Fraud, Waste, and Abuse

OIG, in DHHS, is responsible for investigating instances of fraud, waste, and abuse in the Medicare and Medicaid programs. OIG concentrates its efforts in the following areas:

- Conducting investigations of specific providers suspected of fraud, waste, or abuse for purposes of determining whether criminal, civil, or administrative remedies are warranted;
- Conducting audits, special analyses, and reviews for purposes of discovering and documenting Medicare and Medicaid policy and procedural weaknesses contributing to fraud, waste, or abuse, and making recommendations for corrections;
- Conducting reviews and special projects to determine the level of effort and performance in health provider fraud and abuse control;
- Participating in a program of external communications to inform the health care community, the Congress, other interested organizations, and the public of OIG's concerns and activities related to health care financing integrity;
- Collecting and analyzing Medicare contractor and State Medicaid agency-produced information on resources and results; and
- Participating with other Government agencies and private health insurers in special programs to share techniques and knowledge on preventing health care provider fraud and abuse.

M

Sample State Law: Prohibited Referrals

CO ST § 26-4-410.5
West's Colorado Revised Statutes Annotated
Title 26 Human Services Code
Article 4 Colorado Medical Assistance Act
Part 4 Administrative Procedures

PROVIDERS/PHYSICIANS— PROHIBITION OF CERTAIN REFERRALS

(1) As used in this section, unless the context otherwise requires:

(a) "Financial relationship" means ownership or investment interest in an entity furnishing health services or a compensation arrangement between the physician or an immediate family member of the physician and the entity. An ownership or investment interest may be reflected in equity, debt, or other instruments.

(b) "Immediate family member of the physician" means any spouse, natural or adoptive parent, natural or adoptive child, stepparent, stepchild, stepbrother, stepsister, in-law, grandparent, or grandchild of the physician.

(c) "Physician" means a doctor of medicine or osteopathy, doctor of dental surgery or of dental medicine, doctor of podiatric medicine, doctor of optometry, or chiropractor who is licensed pursuant to title 12, CRS.

(2) Except as provided in subsection (4) of this section, physicians enrolled in the medical assistance program are prohibited from making a referral to an entity for the furnishing of the following health services if the physician or an immediate family member of the physician has a financial relationship with the entity:

(a) Clinical laboratory services;

(b) Physical therapy services;

(c) Occupational therapy services;

(d) Radiology and other diagnostic services;

(e) Radiation therapy services;

(f) Durable medical equipment;

(g) Parenteral or enteral nutrients, equipment, and supplies;

(h) Prosthetics, orthotics, and prosthetic devices;

(i) Home health services;

(j) Outpatient prescription drugs; and

(k) Inpatient and outpatient hospital services.

(3) Any entity that provides the health services identified in subsection (2) of this section as a result of a prohibited referral shall not present a claim.

N

Florida Regulations: Use of Aides in Occupational Therapy

Rule 64B11-4.002, FAC
Fla. Admin. Code Ann. r. 64B11-4.002
Florida Administrative Code Annotated
Title 64 Department of Health
Subtitle 64b11. Occupational Therapy Board
Chapter 64b11-4. Occupational Therapy
Council-Standards of Practice
Current through September 1, 1999

64B11-4.002 OCCUPATIONAL THERAPY AIDES AND OTHER UNLICENSED PERSONNEL INVOLVED IN THE PRACTICE OF OCCUPATIONAL THERAPY

(1) An Occupational therapy aide is an unlicensed person who assists in the practice of occupational therapy, who works under the direct supervision of a licensed occupational therapist of occupational therapy assistant and whose activities require an understanding of occupational therapy but do not require professional of advanced training in the basic anatomical, biological, psychological, and social sciences involved in the practice of occupational therapy. An occupational therapy aide is a worker who is trained on the job to provide supportive services to occupational therapists and occupational therapy assistants. The term occupational therapy aide as used in this section means any unlicensed personnel involved in the practice of occupational therapy.

(2) A licensed occupational therapist or occupational therapy assistant may delegate to occupational therapy aides only specific tasks which are neither evaluative, assessive, task selective nor recommending in nature, and only after insuring that the aide has been appropriately trained for the performance of the task. All delegated patient related tasks must be carried out under direct supervision, which means that the aide must be within the line of vision of the supervising occupational therapist or occupational therapy assistant.

(3) Any duties assigned to an occupational therapy aide must be determined and appropriately supervised by a licensed occupational therapist or occupational therapy assistant and must not exceed the level of training, knowledge, skill, and competence of the individual being supervised. The licensed occupational therapist or occupational therapy assistant is totally and wholly responsible for the acts or actions performed by any occupational therapy aide functioning in the occupational therapy setting.

(4) Occupational therapy aides may perform ministerial duties, tasks and functions without direct supervision which shall include, but not be limited to:

(a) Clerical or secretarial activities

(b) Transportation of patients/clients

(c) Preparing, maintaining or setting up of treatment equipment and work area

(d) Taking care of patients'/clients' personal needs during treatment

(5) Occupational therapy aides shall not perform tasks that are either evaluative, assessive, task selective or recommending in nature which shall include, but not be limited to:

(a) Interpret referrals or prescriptions for occupational therapy services

(b) Perform evaluative procedures

(c) Develop, plan, adjust, or modify treatment procedures

(d) Act on behalf of the occupational therapist in any matter related to direct patient care which requires judgment or decision making except when an emergency condition exists

(e) Act independently or without direct supervision of an occupational therapist

(f) Patient treatment

(g) Any activities which an occupational therapy aide has not demonstrated competence in performing

Florida Regulations: General Supervision of PTAs and Delegation to Unlicensed Personnel by the PT

64 FL ADC 64B176.002
Rule 64B176.002, FAC
Fla. Admin. Code Ann. r. 64B176.002
Florida Administrative Code Annotated
Title 64 Department of Health
Subtitle 64b17 Board of Physical Therapy Practice
Chapter 64b176 Minimum Standards of Practice

64B176.002 GENERAL SUPERVISION OF PHYSICAL THERAPIST ASSISTANTS; ELIGIBILITY; REQUIREMENTS

A physical therapist assistant employed by a board certified orthopedic physician or physiatrist, or a chiropractic physician certified in physiotherapy, shall be under the general supervision of a physical therapist. A physical therapist assistant employed by any physician other than a board certified orthopedic physician or physiatrist or a chiropractic physician certified in physiotherapy shall be under the on-site supervision of a physical therapist. In order to insure adequate supervision of the physical therapist assistant by the supervising physical therapist where general supervision is permitted, there shall be an agreement between the board certified orthopedic physi-

cian or physiatrist or chiropractic physician and the supervising physical therapist, which includes at least the minimum standards of physical therapy practice contained in Rule 64B176.001. The physical therapist assistant shall report all untoward patient responses, inquiries regarding patient prognosis, or the discontinuation of any treatment procedure, to the physical therapist and the board certified orthopedic physician or physiatrist or chiropractic physician certified in physiotherapy.

64 FL ADC 64B176.007
Rule 64B176.007, FAC
Fla. Admin. Code Ann. r. 64B176.007
Florida Administrative Code Annotated
Title 64 Department of Health
Subtitle 64b17 Board of Physical Therapy Practice
Chapter 64b176 Minimum Standards of Practice

64B176.007 DELEGATION TO UNLICENSED PERSONNEL BY THE PHYSICAL THERAPIST

(1) Unlicensed personnel may be utilized to assist in the delivery of patient care treatment by the physical therapist, with direct supervision by the

physical therapist or the physical therapist assistant.

(2) It is the sole responsibility of the physical therapist to consider the task delegated, select the appropriately trained personnel to perform the task, communicate the task or activity desired of the unlicensed personnel, verify the understanding by the unlicensed personnel chosen for the task or activity, and establish procedures for the monitoring of the tasks or activities delegated.

(3) The physical therapist shall retain ultimate responsibility for the patient's physical therapy treatment. Any delegation of treatment to supportive personnel shall be done with consideration of the education, training, and experience of the support personnel. It is the sole responsibility of the physical therapist to define and delineate the education, training, and experience required to perform duties within the physical therapy practice setting, in writing as a part of the practice policies and procedures.

(a) Education entails a technical or professional degree or certification in a specific practice area providing for background and experience.

(b) Qualification by training is the learning of tasks performed and delegated to individuals within the physical therapy practice.

1. The physical therapist shall define the procedures to be used to train unlicensed personnel to perform patient care related tasks or activities within the practice.
2. It is the responsibility of the physical therapist to insure that the necessary training occurred prior to the delegation of a patient care task or activity to unlicensed personnel.

(4) Competency is demonstrated ability to carry out specific functions with reasonable skill and safety. It is the responsibility of the physical therapist to assure competency in delegated skills relative to the tasks delegated.

(5) The physical therapist is responsible for the evaluation and reevaluation of the patient's condition as may be necessary throughout the course of treatment to assure for appropriate treatment and any necessary revision of treatment.

(6) The physical therapist shall not delegate:

(a) Those activities that require the special knowledge, judgment, and skills of the physical therapist, which include:

1. The initial evaluation or any subsequent reevaluation of the patient.
2. Interpretations of the initial evaluation or subsequent reevaluation.
3. Establishment or revision of the physical therapy goals.
4. Development or alteration of the plan of care.
5. Evaluation and interpretation of the progress of the patient in relationship to the plan of care.

(b) Those activities that require the special knowledge, judgment, and skills of the physical therapist assistant, which include:

1. Subsequent reassessments of the patient.
2. Assessment of the progress of the patient in relationship to the plan of care.

(c) Patient progress notes. The unlicensed personnel may document tasks and activities of patients during the patient treatment.

(7) Supervision of unlicensed personnel is the provision of guidance or oversight by qualified physical therapists or physical therapist assistants for the accomplishment of any delegated tasks. A physical therapist may only delegate tasks for which he is qualified or legally entitled to perform, and a physical therapist or physical therapist assistant may only supervise those tasks or activities for which the licensee is qualified or legally entitled to perform.

(8) The number of unlicensed personnel participating in patient care tasks or activities at any one given time shall be determined by the physical therapist dependent upon the individual practice setting, and the individual therapeutic needs of the patients supervised by the physical therapist or physical therapist assistant while assuring for quality care of the patients.

P

Florida Disciplinary Rules for OT, PT, Speech Pathology, and Audiology

Occupational Therapy:
64 FL ADC 64B114.003
Rule 64B114.003, FAC
Fla. Admin. Code Ann. r. 64B114.003
Florida Administrative Code Annotated
Title 64 Department of Health
Subtitle 64b11 Occupational Therapy Board
Chapter 64b114 Occupational Therapy Council
Standards of Practice

64B114.003 STANDARDS OF PRACTICE; DISCIPLINE

(1) Purpose. The legislature created the Board to assure protection of the public from persons who do not meet minimum requirements for safe practice or who pose a danger to the public. Pursuant to Section 455.627, F.S., the Board provides within this rule disciplinary guidelines which shall be imposed upon applicants or licensees whom it regulates under Part III, Chapter 468, F.S. The purpose of this rule is to notify applicants and licensees of the ranges of penalties which will routinely be imposed unless the Board finds it necessary to deviate from the guidelines for the stated reasons given within this rule. The ranges of penalties provided below are based upon a single count violation of each provision listed; multiple counts of the violated provisions or a combina-tion of the violations may result in a higher penalty than that for a single, isolated violation. Each range includes the lowest and highest penalty and all penalties falling between. The purposes of the impo-sition of discipline are to punish the applicants or licensees for violations and to deter them from future violations; to offer opportunities for rehabilitation, when appropriate; and to deter other applicants or licensees from violations.

(2) Among the range of punishments in increas-ing severity are:

(a) Reprimand and a minimum administrative fine of $100.

(b) Probation with conditions to include limita-tions on the type of practice or practice setting, requirement of supervision by a licensee of the Board, employer and self reports, periodic appear-ances before the Board, counseling or participation in the Physician's Recovery Network, payment of administrative fines, and such conditions to assure protection of the public.

(c) Suspension for a minimum of ninety days and thereafter until the licensee appears before the Board to demonstrate current competency and abili-ty to practice safely and compliance with any previ-ous Board orders.

(d) Denial of licensure with conditions to be met prior to any reapplication.

(e) Permanent Revocation.

(3) Aggravating and Mitigating Circumstances. Based upon consideration of aggravating and mitigating factors present in an individual case, the Board may deviate from the penalties recommended below. The Board shall consider as aggravating or mitigating factors the following:

(a) Exposure of patients or public to injury or potential injury, physical or otherwise; none, slight, severe, or death;

(b) Legal status at the time of the offense; no restraints, or legal constraints;

(c) The number of counts or separate offenses established;

(d) The number of times the same offense or offenses have previously been committed by the licensee or applicant;

(e) The disciplinary history of the applicant or licensee in any jurisdiction and the length of practice;

(f) Pecuniary benefit or self-gain inuring to the applicant or licensee;

(g) Any efforts at rehabilitation, attempts by the licensee to correct or to stop violations, or refusal by the licensee to correct or to stop violations;

(h) Any other relevant mitigating factors.

(4) Violations and Range of Penalties. In imposing discipline upon applicants and licensees, in proceedings pursuant to Section 120.57(1) and (2), F.S., the Board shall act in accordance with the following disciplinary guidelines and shall impose a penalty within the range corresponding to the violations set forth below. The verbal identification of offenses are descriptive only; the full language of each statutory provision cited must be consulted in order to determine the conduct included.

VIOLATION—RECOMMENDED RANGE OF PENALTY

(a) Attempting to obtain a license or certificate by bribery, fraud or through an error of the Department or the Board (468.217(1)(a), F.S.). (a) From denial or revocation of license with ability to reapply upon payment of a fine from a minimum of $250 to $1,000.00 to denial of license without ability to reapply.

(b) Action taken against license by another jurisdiction (468.217(1)(b), F.S.). (b) From imposition of discipline comparable to the discipline which would have been imposed if the substantive violation occurred in Florida to suspension or denial of the license until the license is unencumbered in the jurisdiction in which disciplinary action was originally taken, and an administrative fine ranging from $100.00 to $1,000.00. Impaired practitioners working in this state may be ordered into the PRN.

(c) Guilt of crime directly relating to practice or ability to practice (468.217(1)(c), F.S.). (c) From a minimum of six months probation with conditions to revocation or denial of the license and an administrative fine ranging from $100.00 to $1,000.00. Any Board ordered probation shall be for no less time than Court ordered sanctions.

(d) False, deceptive, or misleading advertising(468.217(1)(d), F.S.). (d) From reprimand to one year suspension or denial, and an administrative fine from $250.00 to $1,000.00.

(e) Advertising, practicing under a name other than one's own name (468.217(1)(e), F.S.). (e) From a reprimand to one year suspension or denial, and an administrative fine from $100.00 to $1,000.00.

(f) Failure to report another licensee in violation (468.217(1)(f), F.S.). (f) From reprimand to a minimum of six months probation with conditions or denial, and an administrative fine from $100.00 to $1,000.00.

(g) Aiding unlicensed practice (468.217(1)(g), F.S.). (g) From a minimum of one year probation with conditions to revocation or denial, and an administrative fine from $250.00 to $1,000.00.

(h) Failure to perform legal obligation (468.217(1)(h), F.S.). (h) From a reprimand to revocation or denial, and an administrative fine from $100.00 to $1,000.00.

(i) Filing a false report or failing to file a report as required (468.217(1)(i), F.S.).(i) From one year probation with conditions to revocation or denial, and an administrative fine from $100.00 to $1,000.00.

(j) Kickbacks or split fee arrangements (468.217(1)(j), F.S.). (j) From six months suspension followed by at least one year probation with conditions to revocation or denial, and administrative fine from $250.00 to $1,000.00.

(k) Exercising influence to engage patient in sex (468.217(1)(k), F.S.). (k) From one year suspension followed by at least one year probation with conditions and possible referral to the PRN to revocation or denial, and an administrative fine from $500.00 to $1,000.00.

(l) Deceptive, untrue, or fraudulent representations in the practice of medicine (468.217(1)(l), F.S.). (l) From a minimum of one year probation with conditions to revocation or denial, and an administrative fine from $250.00 to $1,000.00.

(m) Improper solicitation of patients (468.217(1)(m), F.S.). (m) From a minimum of one year probation with conditions to revocation or denial, and an administrative fine from $250.00 to $1,000.00.

(n) Failure to keep written medical records (468.217(1)(n), F.S.). (n) From a reprimand to denial or one year suspension, followed by a minimum of one year probation with conditions and an administrative fine from $100.00 to $1,000.00.

(o) Exercising influence on patient for financial gain (468.217(1)(o), F.S.). (o) From a minimum of one year probation with conditions to denial, and an administrative fine from $250.00 to $1,000.00.

(p) Performing professional services not authorized by patient (468.217(1)(p), F.S.). (p) From a reprimand to denial or one year suspension, followed by a minimum of one year probation with conditions and an administrative fine from $100.00 to $1,000.00.

(q) Malpractice (468.217(1)(q), F.S.). (q) From one year probation with conditions to revocation or denial, and an administrative fine from $150.00 to $1,000.00.

(r) Performing of experimental treatment without informed consent (468.217(1)(r), F.S.). (r) From one year suspension followed by a minimum of one year probation with conditions or denial, and an administrative fine from $250.00 to $1,000.00.

(s) Practicing beyond scope permitted (468.217(1)(s), F.S.). (s) From reprimand to revocation or denial, and an administrative fine from $100.00 to $1,000.00.

(t) Inability to practice occupational therapy with skill and safety (468.217(1)(t), F.S.). (t) From submission of a mental or physical examination directed towards the problem, one year conditions,

possible probation with referral to PRN to revocation or denial, and an administrative fine from $100.00 to $1,000.00.

(u) Delegation of professional responsibilities to an unqualified person (468.217(1)(u), F.S.). (u) From one year probation with conditions to denial or revocation and an administrative fine from $250.00 to $1,000.00.

(v) Violation of law, rule, order, or failure to comply with subpoena (468.217(1)(v), F.S.). (v) From a reprimand to revocation or denial, and an administrative fine from $100.00 to $1,000.00. For failure to comply with subpoena, $250.00 minimum fine and ninety day suspension and thereafter until compliance.

(w) Conspiring to restrict another from lawfully advertising services (468.217(1)(w), F.S.). (w) From a reprimand and an administrative fine from $100.00 to $1,000.00.

(x) False representation of registration (468.223(1), F.S.). (x) From a reprimand to revocation or denial, and an administrative fine from $100.00 to $1,000.00.

(y) Unlicensed practice (468.207, F.S.). (y) A reprimand to revocation or denial, and an administrative fine from $100.00 plus $10 per day for each day over ten worked to $1,000.00.

(5) Stipulations or Settlements. The provisions of this rule are not intended and shall not be construed to limit the ability of the Board to dispose informally of disciplinary actions by stipulation, agreed settlement, or consent order pursuant to Section 120.57(3), F.S.

(6) Letters of Guidance. The provisions of this rule cannot and shall not be construed to limit the authority of the probable cause panel of the Board to direct the Department to send a letter of guidance pursuant to Section 455.621(3), F.S., in any case for which it finds such action appropriate.

(7) Other Action. The provisions of this rule are not intended to and shall not be construed to limit the ability of the Board to pursue or recommend that the Department pursue collateral civil or criminal actions when appropriate.

Q

Internet Resources for Additional Information

LICENSURE

Speech & Language Pathology Licensure Law, Fl Stat § 468.1105-468.1315 (entire text of Florida law):
http://www.leg.state.fl.us/citizen/documents/statutes/1998/ch0468/part01.htm

To find your own state licensure law or search for any state's law, go to *State Legislation* at the link below, find the link to your state, and search your state statutes by keywords:
http://www.washlaw.edu/searchlaw.html

LEGAL SOURCES

Code of Federal Regulations:
http://access.gpo.gov/nara/cfr/cfr-table-search.html

Discrimination laws:
http://www.eeoc.gov

Disability rights laws:
http://www.usdoj.gov

Family Educational Rights and Privacy Act, IDEA regulations, and links to other education-related regulations:
http://www.lrp.com/ed

Federal Register:
http://www.gpo.gov/su_docs/aces/aces140.html

Findlaw-legal search by subject:
http://findlaw.com

Internet law library, US state and territorial law:
http://law.com/lawnet

WashLaw Web (links to law sources):
http://www.washlaw.edu/searchlaw.html

WashLaw Web (links to search engines for case law, federal laws, state laws, and others):
http://www.washlaw.edu/freelib.htm

ETHICS

American Medical Specialty Organization:
http://www.amso.com/ethics.html

Association for Practical and Professional Ethics (links to other ethics resources on the Internet):
http://php.ucs.indiana.edu/~appe/links.html

Bioethics for beginners:
http://www.med.upenn.edu/~bioethic/outreach/bioforbegin/index1.html

Codes of ethics on-line (Healthcare, Center for the Study of Ethics in the Professions, Illinois Institute of Technology):
http://csep.iit.edu/codes/health.html

Bioethics-an introduction:
http://www.med.upenn.edu/~bioethic/outreach/bioforbegin/beginners.html

Ethics on the World Wide Web:
http://commfaculty.fullerton.edu/lester/ethics/ethics_list.html

Ethics on the World Wide Web-Medical ethics:
http://commfaculty.fullerton.edu/lester/ethics/medical.html

Ethics updates (updates on current literature in ethics with many links to ethical theory, applied ethics, and others):
http://ethics.acusd.edu/index.html

Ethics updates glossary:
http://acusd.edu/Glossary.html

Ethics update: a guide to using the World Wide Web in ethics teaching and research (with many links):
http://acusd.edu/resources.html

Grateful Med Bioethicsline search engine:
http://igm.nlm.nih.gov/cgi-bin/doler?account=++&password=++&datafile=bioethicsline

University of British Columbia Centre of Applied Ethics (links to ethical/moral decision making):
http://www.ethics.ubc.ca/resources/dec-mkg

University of British Columbia Centre of Applied Ethics (links to biomedical and health care resources on the World Wide Web):
http://www.ethics.ubc.ca/resources/biomed

University of Minnesota Center for Bioethics:
http://www.med.umn.edu/bioethics/links

University of Pennsylvania Center for Bioethics virtual library:
http://www.med.upenn.edu/~bioethic/outreach/bioforbegin/resources.html

University of Washington School of Medicine (ethics in medicine):
http://edserv.hscer.washington.edu/bioethics

MANAGED CARE

American College of Physicians, Managed Care-frequently asked questions:
http://www.acponline.org/mgdcare/mgdcafaq.htm

American College of Physicians, Managed Care Resources-resources for internists:
http://www.acponline.org/mgdcare/refers.htm

Definitions of managed care terms:
http://www.amso.com/terms.html

Disabilities and managed care:
http://managedcare.hhs.gov/

Florida Managed Care Institute national news:
http://fmciweb.com/nationalnews.htm

The HMO Page:
http://www.hmopage.org

The Institute for Managed Care at Michigan State University links:
http://healthteam.msu.edu/links.htm

Managed care daily briefing:
http://www.managedcaremag.com/

Managed care on-line:
http://www.mcol.com/online.htm

Managed care resources (including links to government sites, papers, and publications):
http://www.chcs.org/resources.htm

The Medicaid managed care program:
http://www.chcs.org/pdf/CHCS/pdf
Overview of managed care:
http://www.wnet.org/archive/mhc/Overview/essay.html

ADDITIONAL RESOURCES

Barbara L. Kornblau's webpage:
http://www.nova.edu/~kornblau/index.html

Author's comment: Please remember Internet sites change frequently.

R

Bibliography and Additional Sources of Information

LAW

Books

American Occupational Therapy Association. (1996). *The occupational therapy manager.* Bethesda, MD: AOTA.

Areen, J., King, P. A., Goldberg, S., Gostin, L., & Capron, A. M. (1996). *Law, medicine & science.* Westbury, NY: Foundation Press.

Biano, E. A., & Hirsh, H. L. (1995). Consent to and refusal of medical treatment. In Sanbar, S. (Ed.). *Legal medicine.* St. Louis: Mosby.

(1979). *Black's law dictionary* (5th ed.). St. Paul, MN: West Publishing.

Calloway, S. (1985). *Nursing and the law.* Eau Clare, WI: Professional Education Systems.

Ellexson, M. T., & Kornblau, B. L. (1995). Reasonable accommodations: the process. In Isernhagen, S. (Ed.). *Work injury: the full spectrum of management.* Gaithersburg, MD: Aspen.

Equal Employment Opportunity Commission. (1992). *Technical assistance manual to Title I of the Americans With Disabilities Act.* Washington, DC: US Government Printing Office.

Greenwood, J. G., & Wyman, E. T. (1997). The workers' compensation system. In Nordin, M., Andersson, G. B., & Pope, M. H. (Eds.). *Musculoskeletal disorders in the workplace.* St. Louis: Mosby.

Himmelstein, J., Pransky, G., & Fram, D. (1997). Preemployment and pre-placement evaluations and the Americans With Disabilities Act. In Nordin, M., Andersson, G. B., & Pope, M. H. (Eds.). *Musculoskeletal disorders in the workplace.* St. Louis: Mosby.

Hopkins, B. R., & Anderson, B. S. (1990). *The counselor and the law.* Alexandria, VA: American Association for Counseling and Development.

Kornblau, B. L. (1998). Health care ergonomics and the American With Disabilities Act. In Rice, V. *Clinical ergonomics.* Boston: Butterworth-Heinemann.

Kornblau, B. L. (1998). The Americans With Disabilities Act: legal ramifications of ADA consultation. In Rice, V. *Clinical ergonomics.* Boston: Butterworth-Heinemann.

Leger, D., & Kemp, J. D. (1997). The Americans With Disabilities Act. In Nordin, M., Andersson, G. B., & Pope, M. H. (Eds.). *Musculoskeletal disorders in the workplace.* St. Louis: Mosby.

MacDonald, M. G., Meyer, K. C., & Essig, B. (1985). *Health care law: a practical guide.* New York: Matthew Bender and Associates.

Petrocelli, W., & Repa, B. K. (1995). *Sexual harassment on the job.* Berkeley, CA: Nolo Press.

Prosser, W. L. (1971). *Law of torts.* St. Paul, MN: West Publishing.

Reamer, F. G. (1991). AIDS & ethics. New York: Columbia University Press.

Romano, J. L. (1998). *Legal rights of the catastrophically ill and injured: a family guide.* Norristown, PA: Author.

Rosenblatt, R. E., Law, S. A., & Rosenbaum, S. (1997). *Law and the American health care system.* Westbury, NY: Foundation Press.

Sanbar, S. (Ed.) (1995). *Legal medicine.* St. Louis: Mosby.

Scott, R. W. (1997). *Promoting legal awareness in physical and occupational therapy.* St. Louis: Mosby.

Spieler, E. (1995). Legal issues in occupational medicine. In Herrington ,T. N., & Moorse, L. H. (Eds.). *Occupational injuries, evaluation, management, and prevention.* St. Louis: Mosby.

Stromberg, C., Hagarty, D. J., & Geibenluft, R. F., et. al. (1988). The psychologist's legal *handbook*. Washington, DC: Council for National Register of Health Service Providers in Psychology.

Wings, K. R. (1995). *The law and the public's health.* Ann Arbor, MI: Health Association Press.

Weinstein, M. M. (1991). *The law of federal income taxation.* Deerfield, IL: Callaghan and Company.

Journal Articles

Barber, T. (1998). Beyond noncompete agreements: using Florida's Trade Secrets Act to prevent former employees from disclosing sensitive information to competitors. *Florida Bar Journal*, 72.

Bisbee, H. R. (1998). The art of licensure. *Florida Bar Journal*, 72.

Blumstein, J. F. (1996). The fraud and abuse statute in an evolving health care marketplace: life in a health care speakeasy. *American Journal of Law & Medicine, 22,* 205-231.

Bucy, P. H. (1996). Crimes by health care providers. *University of Illinois Review, 5,* 89.

Darken, K. J. (1997). Understanding the new federal health care fraud legislation. *Florida Bar Journal*, 71.

Ellis, D. R. (1998). Cyberlaw and computer technology: a primer on the law of intellectual property protection. *Florida Bar Journal*, 72.

Greaney, T. L. (1997). Night landings on an aircraft carrier: hospital mergers and antitrust law. *American Journal of Law & Medicine*, 23.

Kornblau, B. L., & Ellexson, M. T. (1993). Managing workers' compensation with pre-placement screening. *The Journal of Workers' Compensation*, 2.

Makar, M. C. (1996). Nursing in Florida: the path to professional liability. *Fla B J*, 70.

O'Leary, H., & Imperato, G. (1991). Defending a health care provider in a criminal fraud investigation. *Florida Bar Journal, 65.*

Ranke, B. A. , & Moriarty, M. P. (1997). An overview of professional liability in occupational therapy. *American Journal of Occupational Therapy, 51, 671.*

Salcido, R. (1996). Applications of the False Claims Act: Knowledge: Standard: What one must know to be held liable under the Act. *The Heath Lawyer, 8,* 1.

Stromberg, C., Loeb, L., Thomen, S., & Krause, J. (1993). Malpractice and other professional liability-the psychologist's legal update. *National Register of Health Service Providers in Psychology, 3, 1-15.*

Stancliff, B. L. (1997). Invisible victims. *Occupational Therapy Practice, 2, 19.*

Cases

Arizona v. Maricopa County Medical Society, 457 U.S. 332 (1982)

Board of Regents v. Taborsky, 648 So. 2d 748 (Fla. 2d DCA 1994)

Northern Pacific Railway v. United States, 365 U.S. 1, 4-5 (1958)

Statutes and Regulations

ADA § 102(b)(5)

The Age Discrimination in Employment Act of 1967 (Pub. L. 90-202)

American With Disabilities Act of 1990, 42 USC §§ 12101-12113, 1992

Fair Housing Act, 42 USC § 2601 et seq.

Family Educational Rights and Privacy Act, 20 USCA § 1232g & h, (1974) (FERPA) Family Medical Leave Act, 29 USC §§ 2601-2619, 1993

Fla Stat § 688.002(4)

Fla Stat § 688.003(1)

Fla Stat § 812.081

Department of Health and Human Services, Regulations on Protection of Human Services, 45 CFR 46 (1994)

Health Care Portability and Accountability Act of 1996, Public Law 104-191 (1996)

Health Insurance Manual for Home Health Care § 106.1 7/92 (HCFA)

Omnibus Budget Reconciliation Act of 1987, Pub. L. No. 100-203, 101 Stat. 1330 (OBRA)

28 CFR 36 §102

28 CFR 36 §104

Appendix to 29 CFR 14, (a), Interpretive Guidelines

29 CFR §1604.11a

29 CFR § 1630(2)(g)

29 CFR § 1630.2(m); Americans with Disabilities Act § 101(8)

29 CFR §1630.2(o)

34 CFR § 99

ETHICS

Books

American Occupational Therapy Association. (1998). *Reference guide to the occupational therapy code of ethics.* Bethesda, MD: AOTA.

Areen, J., King, P. A., Goldberg, S., Gostin, L., & Capron, A. M. (1996). *Law, medicine & science.* Westbury, NY: Foundation Press.

Beauchamp, T. L., & Childress, J. F. (1994). *Principles of biomedical ethics.* New York: Oxford University Press.

Biano, E. A., & Hirsh, H. L. (1995). Consent to and refusal of medical treatment. In Sanbar, S. (Ed.). *Legal medicine.* St. Louis: Mosby.

Gert, B., Culver, C. M., & Clouser, K. D. (1997). *Bioethics: a return to fundamentals.* New York: Oxford University Press.

Hansen, R. A. (1992). Ethical considerations for the consultant. In Jaffe, E. G., & Epstein, C. F. (Eds.). *Occupational therapy consultation: theories, principles and practice.* St. Louis: Mosby.

Monagle, J. F., & Thomasma, D. C. (1998). *Health care ethics.* Gaithersburg, MD: Aspen.

Purtillo, R. (1993). *Ethical dimensions in the health professions.* Philadelphia: Saunders.

Shannon, T. A. (1997). *An introduction to bioethics.* New York: Paulist Press.

Shannon, T. A. (Ed.) (1993). *Bioethics.* New York: Paulist Press.

Sim, J. (1997). *Ethical decision making in practice.* Oxford, UK: Butterworth Heinemann.

Stromberg, C., et al. (1988). *The psychologist's legal handbook.* Washington, DC: Council for National Register of Health Service Providers in Psychology.

Taylor, P. W. (1975). *Principles of ethics: an introduction.* Encino, CA: Dickenson Publishing Company.

Weston, A. (1997). *A practical companion to ethics.* New York: Oxford University Press.

Journals

American Journal of Law & Medicine

Hastings Center Report

The Journal of Law, Medicine & Ethics

Journal Articles

Dickens, B. D. (1995). Conflicts of interest in Canadian health care law. *American Journal of Law & Medicine,* 22.

Rodwin, M. A. (1995). Strains in the fiduciary metaphor: divided loyalties and obligations in a changing health care system. *American Journal of Law & Medicine,* 22.

Watson, S. D. (1995). Medicaid physician participation: patients, poverty, and physicians' self-interest. *American Journal of Law & Medicine,* 22.

Cases

Hammonds v. Aetna Casualty & Surety Co., 243 F.Supp 793 (N.D. Ohio 1965)

MANAGED CARE

Books

American Occupational Therapy Association. (1996). *Managed care: an occupational therapy sourcebook.* Bethesda, MD: AOTA.

American Occupational Therapy Association. (1996). *The occupational therapy manager.* Bethesda, MD: AOTA.

Baldor, R. A. (1996). *Managed care made simple.* Cambridge, MA: Blackwell Science.

Christensen, K. T. (1998). Ethically important decisions in managed care organizations. In Monagle, J. F., & Thomasma, D. C. *Health care ethics.* Gaithersburg, MD: Aspen.

DeMarco, W. J., & Wolfe, K. (1995). Managed care concepts in the delivery of disability management: services to industry. In Shrey, D. E., & Lecerte, M. (Eds.). *Principle and Practices of disability management in industry.* Winter Park, FL: GR Press.

Numbers, R. L. (1979). The third party: health insurance in America. In Vogel, M. J., & Rosenberg. *The therapeutic revolution: essays in the social history of American medicine.* Philadelphia: University of Pennsylvania Press.

Pellegrino, E. D. (1998). Rationing health care: the ethics of medical gatekeeping. In Monagle, J. F., & Thomasma, D. C. *Health care ethics.* Gaithersburg, MD: Aspen.

Rosenblatt, R. E., Law, S. A., & Rosenbaum, S. (1997). *Law and the American health care system.* Westbury, NY: Foundation Press.

Sanbar, S. (Ed.) (1995). *Legal medicine.* St. Louis: Mosby.

Stromberg, C., et al. (1988). *The psychologist's legal handbook.* Washington, DC: Council for National Register of Health Service Providers in Psychology.

Sultz, H. A., & Young, K. M. (1988). *Health care USA: understanding its organization and delivery.* Gaithersburg, MD: Aspen.

Journal Articles

Dickens, B. D. (1995). Conflicts of interest in Canadian health care law. *American Journal of Law & Medicine,* 22.

Burton, D. N., & Popok, M. S. (1998). Managed care 101. *Florida Bar Journal,* 72.

Farrell, M. G. (1997). ERISA preemption and regulation of managed health care: the case for managed federalism. *American Journal of Law & Medicine,* 23.

Few, A., & Trezevant, J. G. (1998). Fighting the battle against health care fraud: federal enforcement actions. *Florida Bar Journal,* 72.

Grossman, A. R., & Rock, R. A. (1998). Fee splitting and the management of medical practices: a history of board of medicine declaratory statements. *Florida Bar Journal,* 72.

Gunderson, M. (1997). Eliminating conflicts of managed care organizations through disclosure and consent. *Journal of Law, Medicine & Ethics,* 25, 92-98.

Hashimoto, D. M. (1996). The future role of managed care and capitation in workers' compensation. *American Journal of Law & Medicine,* 22.

Latham, S. R. (1996). Regulation of incentive payments to physicians. *American Journal of Law & Medicine,* 22.

Lockman, S. M., & Silverman, T. E. (1998). Formation of hybrid type organizations: virtual mergers of health care systems. *Florida Bar Journal,* 72.

Malinowski, M. J. (1996). Capitation, advance in medical technology, and the advent of a new era in medical ethics. *American Journal of Law & Medicine,* 22.

Martin, J. A., & Bjerknes, L. K. (1996). The legal and ethical implications of gag clauses in physician contracts. *American Journal of Law & Medicine, 22.*

Rodwin, M. A. (1995). Strains in the fiduciary metaphor: divided loyalties and obligations in a changing health care system. *American Journal of Law & Medicine, 22.*

Stromberg, C., Loeb, L., Thomen, S., & Krause, J. (1996). State initiatives in health care reform-the psychologist's legal update. *National Register of Health Service Providers in Psychology, 8.*

Stromberg, C., Loeb, L., Thomen, S., & Krause, J. (1997).

Surviving the minefields of managed care contracting-the psychologist's legal update. *National Register of Health Service Providers in Psychology, 9.*

Watson, S. D. (1995). Medicaid physician participation: patients, poverty, and physicians' self-interest. *American Journal of Law & Medicine, 22.*

Weiner, J., & de Lissovoy, G. (1993). Razing the Tower of Babel: a taxonomy for managed care and health insurance plans. *Journal of Health Politics, Policy and Law, 75, 18.*

APPENDIX

S

A Guide to Disability Rights Laws

US Department of Justice
Civil Rights Division
Disability Rights Section
A Guide to Disability Rights Laws
October 1, 1996

CONTENTS

This guide provides an overview of Federal civil rights laws that ensure equal opportunity for people with disabilities. To find out more about how these laws may apply to you, contact the agencies and organizations listed below.

AMERICANS WITH DISABILITIES ACT (ADA)

The ADA prohibits discrimination on the basis of disability in employment, State and local government, public accommodations, commercial facilities, transportation, and telecommunications. It also applies to the United States Congress.

To be protected by the ADA, one must have a disability or have a relationship or association with an individual with a disability. An individual with a disability is defined by the ADA as a person who has a physical or mental impairment that substantially limits one or more major life activities, a person who has a history or record of such an impairment, or a person who is perceived by others as having such an impairment. The ADA does not specifically name all of the impairments that are covered.

ADA Title I: Employment

Title I requires employers with 15 or more employees to provide qualified individuals with disabilities an equal opportunity to benefit from the full range of employment-related opportunities available to others. For example, it prohibits discrimination in recruitment, hiring, promotions, training, pay, social activities, and other privileges of employment. It restricts questions that can be asked about an applicant's disability before a job offer is made, and it requires that employers make reasonable accommodation to the known physical or mental limitations of otherwise qualified individuals with disabilities, unless it results in undue hardship. Religious entities with 15 or more employees are covered under Title I.

Title I complaints must be filed with the U.S. Equal Employment Opportunity Commission (EEOC) within 180 days of the date of discrimination, or 300 days if the charge is filed with a designated State or local fair employment practice agency. Individuals may file a lawsuit in Federal court only after they receive a "right-to-sue" letter from the EEOC.

Charges of employment discrimination on the basis of disability may be filed at any U.S. Equal Employment Opportunity Commission field office. Field offices are located in 50 cities throughout the U.S. and are listed in most telephone directories under "U.S. Government."

For the appropriate EEOC field office in your geographic area, call:

(800) 669-4000 (voice)
(800) 669-6820 (TDD)

Information on EEOC-enforced laws may be obtained by calling:

(800) 669-EEOC (voice)
(800) 800-3302 (TDD)

For information on how to accommodate a specific individual with a disability, call the Job Accommodation Network at:

(800) 526-7234 (voice/TDD)
(800) ADA-WORK (voice/TDD)

ADA Title II: State and Local Government Activities

Title II covers all activities of State and local governments regardless of the government entity's size or receipt of Federal funding. Title II requires that State and local governments give people with disabilities an equal opportunity to benefit from all of their programs, services, and activities (e.g., public education, employment, transportation, recreation, health care, social services, courts, voting, and town meetings).

State and local governments are required to follow specific architectural standards in the new construction and alteration of their buildings. They also must relocate programs or otherwise provide access in inaccessible older buildings, and communicate effectively with people who have hearing, vision, or speech disabilities. Public entities are not required to take actions that would result in undue financial and administrative burdens. They are required to make reasonable modifications to policies, practices, and procedures where necessary to avoid discrimination, unless they can demonstrate that doing so would fundamentally alter the nature of the service, program, or activity being provided.

Complaints of Title II violations may be filed with the Department of Justice within 180 days of the date of discrimination. In certain situations, cases may be referred to a mediation program sponsored by the Department. The Department may bring a lawsuit where it has investigated a matter and has been unable to resolve violations.

For more information or to file a complaint, contact:

Disability Rights Section
Civil Rights Division
U.S. Department of Justice
P.O. Box 66738
Washington, D.C. 20035-6738

You may also call for information at:
(800) 514-0301 (voice)
(800) 514-0383 (TDD)

Title II may also be enforced through private lawsuits in Federal court. It is not necessary to file a complaint with the Department of Justice (DOJ) or any other Federal agency, or to receive a "right-to-sue" letter, before going to court.

ADA Title II: Public Transportation

The transportation provisions of Title II cover public transportation services, such as city buses and public rail transit (e.g. subways, commuter rails, Amtrak). Public transportation authorities may not discriminate against people with disabilities in the provision of their services. They must comply with requirements for accessibility in newly purchased vehicles, make good faith efforts to purchase or lease accessible used buses, remanufacture buses in an accessible manner, and, unless it would result in an undue burden, provide paratransit where they operate fixed-route bus or rail systems. Paratransit is a service where individuals who are unable to use the regular transit system independently (because of a physical or mental impairment) are picked up and dropped off at their destinations.

Questions and complaints about public transportation should be directed to:

Federal Transit Administration
U.S. Department of Transportation
400 Seventh Street, S.W.
Washington, D.C. 20590

Documents and questions:
(202) 366-1656 (voice)
(202) 366-4567 (TDD)

Legal questions:
(202) 366-1936 (voice/relay)
(202) 366-9306 (voice)
(202) 755-7687 (TDD)

Complaints and enforcement:
202) 366-2285 (voice)
(202) 366-0153 (TDD)

ADA Title III: Public Accommodations

Title III covers businesses and nonprofit service providers that are public accommodations, privately operated entities offering certain types of courses and examinations, privately operated transportation, and commercial facilities. Public accommodations are private entities who own, lease, lease to, or operate facilities such as restaurants, retail stores, hotels, movie theaters, private schools, convention centers, doctors' offices, homeless shelters, transportation depots, zoos, funeral homes, day care centers, and recreation facilities including sports stadiums and fitness clubs. Transportation services provided by private entities are also covered by Title III.

Public accommodations must comply with basic nondiscrimination requirements that prohibit exclusion, segregation, and unequal treatment. They also must comply with specific requirements related to architectural standards for new and altered buildings; reasonable modifications to policies, practices, and procedures; effective communication with people with hearing, vision, or speech disabilities; and other access requirements. Additionally, public accommodations must remove barriers in existing buildings where it is easy to do so without much difficulty or expense, given the public accommodation's resources.

Courses and examinations related to professional, educational, or trade-related applications, licensing, certifications, or credentialing must be provided in a place and manner accessible to people with disabilities, or alternative accessible arrangements must be offered.

Commercial facilities, such as factories and warehouses, must comply with the ADA's architectural standards for new construction and alterations.

Complaints of Title III violations may be filed with the Department of Justice. In certain situations, cases may be referred to a mediation program sponsored by the Department. The Department is authorized to bring a lawsuit where there is a pattern or practice of discrimination in violation of Title III, or where an act of discrimination raises an issue of general public importance. Title III may also be enforced through private lawsuits. It is not necessary to file a complaint with the Department of Justice (or any Federal agency), or to receive a "right-to-sue" letter, before going to court.

For more information or to file a complaint, contact:

Disability Rights Section
Civil Rights Division
U.S. Department of Justice
P.O. Box 66738
Washington, D.C. 20035-6738

You may also call for information at:
(800) 514-0301 (voice)
(800) 514-0383 (TDD)

ADA Title IV: Telecommunications

Title IV addresses telephone and television access for people with hearing and speech disabilities. It requires common carriers (telephone companies) to establish interstate and intrastate telecommunications relay services (TRS) 24 hours a day, 7 days a week. TRS enables callers with hearing and speech disabilities who use text telephones (TTYs or TDDs), and callers who use voice telephones, to communicate with each other through a third party communications assistant. The Federal Communications Commission (FCC) has set minimum standards for TRS services. Title IV also requires closed captioning of Federally funded public service announcements.

For more information about TRS, contact the FCC at:

Federal Communications Commission
1919 M Street, N.W.
Washington, D.C. 20554

Documents and questions:
(202) 418-0190 (voice)
(202) 418-2555 (TDD)

Legal questions:
(202) 418-2357 (voice)
(202) 418-0484 (TDD)

FAIR HOUSING ACT

The Fair Housing Act, as amended in 1988, prohibits housing discrimination on the basis of race, color, religion, sex, disability, familial status, and national origin. Its coverage includes private housing, housing that receives Federal financial assistance, and State and local government housing. It is unlawful to discriminate in any aspect of selling or renting housing or to deny a dwelling to a buyer or renter because of the disability of that individual, an individual associated with the buyer or renter, or an individual who intends to live in the residence. Other covered activities include, for example, financing, zoning practices, new construction design, and advertising.

The Fair Housing Act requires owners of housing facilities to make reasonable exceptions in their policies and operations to afford people with disabilities equal housing opportunities. For example, a landlord with a "no pets" policy may be required to grant an exception to this rule and allow an individual who is blind to keep a guide dog in the residence. The Fair Housing Act also requires landlords to allow tenants with disabilities to make reasonable access-related modifications to their private living space, as well as to common use spaces. (The landlord is not required to pay for the changes.) The Act further requires that new multifamily housing with four or more units be designed and built to allow access for persons with disabilities. This includes accessible common use areas, doors that are wide enough for wheelchairs, kitchens and bathrooms that allow a person using a wheelchair to maneuver, and other adaptable features within the units.

Complaints of Fair Housing Act violations may be filed with the U.S. Department of Housing and Urban Development.

For more information or to file a complaint, contact:

Office of Program Compliance and Disability Rights
Office of Fair Housing and Equal Opportunity
U.S. Department of Housing and Urban Development
451 7th Street, SW (Room 5242)
Washington, D.C. 20140

You may also call the Fair Housing Information Clearinghouse at:
(800) 343-3442 (voice)
(800) 483-2209 (TDD)

Additionally, the Department of Justice can file cases involving a pattern or practice of discrimination. The Fair Housing Act may also be enforced through private lawsuits.

AIR CARRIER ACCESS ACT

The Air Carrier Access Act prohibits discrimination in air transportation by air carriers against qualified individuals with physical or mental impairments. It applies only to air carriers that provide regularly scheduled services for hire to the public. Requirements address a wide range of issues including boarding assistance and certain accessibility features in newly built aircraft and new or altered airport facilities. People may enforce rights under the Air Carrier Access Act by filing a complaint with the U.S. Department of Transportation, or by bringing a lawsuit in Federal court.

For more information or to file a complaint contact:

Departmental Office of Civil Rights
Office of the Secretary
U.S. Department of Transportation
400 Seventh Street, S.W.
Washington, D.C. 20590
(202) 366-4648 (voice)
(202) 366-8538 (TDD)

You may also contact:
Aviation Consumer Protection Division, C-75
U.S. Department of Transportation
400 Seventh Street, S.W.
Washington, D.C. 20590
(202) 366-2220 (voice)
(202) 755-7687 (TDD)

CIVIL RIGHTS OF INSTITUTIONALIZED PERSONS ACT

The Civil Rights of Institutionalized Persons Act (CRIPA) authorizes the U.S. Attorney General to investigate conditions of confinement at State and local government institutions such as prisons, jails, pretrial detention centers, juvenile correctional facilities, publicly operated nursing homes, and institutions for people with psychiatric or developmental disabilities. Its purpose is to allow the Attorney General to uncover and correct widespread deficiencies that seriously jeopardize the health and safety of residents of institutions. The Attorney General does not have authority under CRIPA to investigate isolated incidents or to represent individual institutionalized persons.

The Attorney General may initiate civil lawsuits where there is reasonable cause to believe that conditions are "egregious or flagrant," that they are subjecting residents to "grievous harm," and that they are part of a "pattern or practice" of resistance to residents' full enjoyment of constitutional or Federal rights, including Title II of the ADA and section 504 of the Rehabilitation Act.

For more information or to bring a matter to the Department of Justice's attention, contact:
Special Litigation Section
Civil Rights Division
U.S. Department of Justice
P.O. Box 66400
Washington, D.C. 20035-6400
(202) 514-6255 (voice/relay)

INDIVIDUALS WITH DISABILITIES EDUCATION ACT

The Individuals with Disabilities Education Act (IDEA) (formerly called P.L. 94-142 or the Education for all Handicapped Children Act of 1975) requires public schools to make available to all eligible children with disabilities a free appropriate public education in the least restrictive environment appropriate to their individual needs.

IDEA requires public school systems to develop appropriate Individualized Education Programs (IEPs) for each child. The specific special education and related services outlined in each IEP reflect the individualized needs of each student.

IDEA also mandates that particular procedures be followed in the development of the IEP. Each student's IEP must be developed by a team of knowledgeable persons and must be at least reviewed annually. The team includes the child's teacher; the parents, subject to certain limited exceptions; the child, if determined appropriate; an agency representative who is qualified to provide or supervise the provision of special education; and other individuals at the parents' or agency's discretion.

If parents disagree with the proposed IEP, they can request a due process hearing and a review from the State educational agency if applicable in that state. They also can appeal the State agency's decision to State or Federal court.

For more information, contact:
Office of Special Education Programs
U.S. Department of Education
330 C Street, S.W. (Room 3086)
Washington, D.C. 20202
(202) 205-5507 (voice)
(202) 205-9754 (TDD)

REHABILITATION ACT

The Rehabilitation Act prohibits discrimination on the basis of disability in programs conducted by Federal agencies, in programs receiving Federal financial assistance, in Federal employment, and in the employment practices of Federal contractors. The standards for determining employment discrimination under the Rehabilitation Act are the same as those used in Title I of the Americans with Disabilities Act.

SECTION 501

Section 501 requires affirmative action and nondiscrimination in employment by Federal agencies of the executive branch. To obtain more information or to file a complaint, employees should contact their agency's Equal Employment Opportunity Office.

SECTION 503

Section 503 requires affirmative action and prohibits employment discrimination by Federal government contractors and subcontractors with contracts of more than $10,000.

For more information on section 503, contact:
Office of Federal Contract Compliance Programs
U.S. Department of Labor
200 Constitution Ave, NW
Washington, D.C. 20210
(202) 219-9423 (voice/relay)

SECTION 504

Section 504 states that "no qualified individual with a disability in the United States shall be excluded from, denied the benefits of, or be subjected to discrimination under" any program or activity that either receives Federal financial assistance or is conducted by any Executive agency or the United States Postal Service.

Each Federal agency has its own set of section 504 regulations that apply to its own programs. Agencies that provide Federal financial assistance also have section 504 regulations covering entities that receive Federal aid. Requirements common to these regulations include reasonable accommodation for employees with disabilities; program accessibility; effective communication with people who have hearing or vision disabilities; and accessible new construction and alterations. Each agency is responsible for enforcing its own regulations. Section 504 may also be enforced through private lawsuits. It is not necessary to file a complaint with a Federal agency or to receive a "right-to-sue" letter before going to court.

For information on how to file 504 complaints with the appropriate agency, contact:
Disability Rights Section
Civil Rights Division
U.S. Department of Justice
P.O. Box 66738
Washington, D.C. 20035-6738
(800) 514-0301 (voice)
(800) 514-0383 (TDD)

ARCHITECTURAL BARRIERS ACT

The Architectural Barriers Act (ABA) requires that buildings and facilities that are designed, constructed, or altered with Federal funds, or leased by a Federal agency, comply with Federal standards for physical accessibility. ABA requirements are limited to architectural standards in new and altered buildings and in newly leased facilities. They do not address the activities conducted in those buildings and facilities. Facilities of the U.S. Postal Service are covered by the ABA.

For more information or to file a complaint, contact:
The U.S. Architectural and Transportation Barriers Compliance Board
1331 F Street, N.W. (Suite 1000)
Washington, D.C. 20004-1111
(800) 872-2253 (voice)
(800) 993-2822 (TDD)

OTHER SOURCES OF DISABILITY RIGHTS INFORMATION

Regional Disability and Business Technical Assistance Centers:
(800) 949-4232 (voice/TDD)

U.S. Department of Justice, Civil Rights Division, Americans with Disabilities Act Internet Home Page:
http://www.usdoj.gov/crt/ada/adahom1.htm

INDEX